CHAIR

YOGA

FOR WEIGHT LOSS

KRISTEN PAYTON

TABLE OF CONTENTS

20 SEATED WALKING WITH A SUPPORT

21 ARMS AND LEGS UNILATERAL STRETCHING

22 LIFTING + LEGS APERTURE

23 ALTERNATE LEGS STRETCHING

24 LEGS UNILATERAL STRETCHING + ARMS LIFT

25 FROG ON THE CHAIR

26 PELVIS ROTATION WHEN SITTING

27 UNILATERAL FORWARD FLEXION

28 UNILATERAL STRETCHING WITH YOUR ARMS AS SUPPORTS

29 LATERAL STRETCHING

30 SWINGS WITH HANDS TOGETHER

31 LATERAL FLEXION

32 SEATED UNILATERAL CRUNCHES

33 UNILATERAL AND COMPLETE STRETCHING

34 BUST FLEXION AND BENDING FORWARD

35 BULGARIAN SQUAT WITH SUPPORT

36 BALLERINAS WITH SUPPORT

37 STANDING SUPERMAN POSE

38 SPINE COMPLETE STRETCHING

39 PRAYING POSE + STRETCHING

40 SHOULDERS ROTATION

IMPORTANT INFORMATION BEFORE YOU START!

28-DAY FAT BURNING PROGRAM

CHAIR YOGA FOR WEIGHT LOSS - INTRODUCTION

WELCOME TO YOUR CHAIR YOGA JOURNEY

I'm so honored to welcome you to this program and grateful you've chosen to take this step toward a stronger, healthier, and more peaceful version of yourself. Chair yoga is not just about physical movement—it's about reclaiming time for your body and your well-being in a way that's gentle, supportive, and deeply empowering.

This practice is designed to meet you exactly where you are—whether you're looking to improve your posture, regain balance, reduce stress, or lose weight in a sustainable, compassionate way. And best of all, you don't need fancy equipment or experience to begin. Just a sturdy chair, a bit of space, and a willingness to show up for yourself.

THE FOUNDATIONS OF CHAIR YOGA

Chair yoga is rooted in the same principles as traditional yoga—balance, breath, flexibility, strength, and presence—but it's modified to be more accessible and adaptable. This discipline embraces your current physical condition and invites in progress, not perfection. Whether you're dealing with joint stiffness, recovering from an injury, or simply prefer a lower-impact approach, chair yoga offers the benefits of movement without the strain.

What makes this practice so powerful is that it connects body and mind through breath, focus, and intention. It's not just about stretching or burning calories—although those things can and do happen. It's about aligning your physical actions with mental clarity, emotional calm, and self-awareness.

In today's fast-paced world, we often move from task to task without taking a moment to check in with ourselves. Chair yoga gives us that moment. Each session becomes an invitation to slow down, breathe deeper, and move with purpose.

A PRACTICE FOR EVERYONE

One of the things I love most about chair yoga is that it's truly inclusive. This is not a program for a certain age group or fitness level—it's for all women who want to move more mindfully and feel better in their bodies. You're not too old. You're not too out of shape. You're not too busy. This is your time, and you're more than ready.

Throughout this book, you'll find a variety of exercises that target different muscle groups and focus areas. I've built in options to modify based on your comfort level, so you can always find a version of the movement that feels safe and effective. There's no rushing, no pressure, and no judgment—only encouragement, support, and steady progress.

MY PERSONAL APPROACH TO THIS BOOK

When I wrote this guide, my top priority was clarity and ease. Each exercise is laid out across two facing pages: on your left, you'll find a step-by-step description of how to perform the move, including how and when to breathe. On your right, you'll see a photo demonstration that shows correct posture, form, and alignment.

But I didn't stop there. I've also recorded a complete video for each exercise so you can follow along visually. These videos are included with your purchase and accessible through a simple QR code printed inside the book. Watching the videos alongside reading the instructions will help you feel confident and safe as you build your practice.

This combination—written steps, visual guides, and video tutorials—creates a 360-degree experience that makes it easier than ever to succeed. You'll never feel like you're guessing or struggling to keep up. I'm right there with you, guiding you through it all.

HOW I SELECTED THE EXERCISES

The movements in this book weren't chosen at random. I carefully curated each one to target key areas of the body while keeping things safe, accessible, and effective. My focus was on exercises that can:

- Support weight loss through gentle calorie burn and muscle activation
- Improve balance and stability to prevent falls and increase confidence
- Build coordination and mind-body awareness
- Increase spinal flexibility and core strength to support posture
- Expand lung capacity and reduce stress through focused breathwork

Each session helps activate the body's natural fat-burning processes while also building strength and flexibility. And because the exercises are designed to be low-impact, they're kind to joints and suitable for daily practice. You'll find that your body responds positively when you move with care and intention.

WHY SPINE HEALTH AND BREATHING MATTER

One of the most important systems we can support through yoga is the spine. Your spine is literally your backbone of your entire physical structure. When it's stiff or tense, you feel it—whether it's in your neck, shoulders, or lower back. That's why I've included a variety of movements focused on spinal decompression, lengthening, and support.

As we release tension from your back and engage the core muscles, posture naturally improves. You'll likely find yourself standing taller, breathing deeper, and feeling more centered.

Speaking of breath—your breath is your greatest tool in this practice. Controlled, mindful breathing helps oxygenate the body, calm the nervous system, and connect each movement with awareness. Breathing well isn't just for yoga—it helps regulate mood, reduce anxiety, and improve focus throughout your day.

SUPPORTING THE AGING BODY WITH GRACE

Our bodies change as we age. Flexibility decreases, muscle mass may decline, and balance can become more fragile. But aging doesn't mean giving up on movement. In fact, movement becomes even more essential.

Chair yoga provides a beautiful and sustainable way to stay strong, flexible, and mobile throughout your life. This book includes specific exercises to stimulate circulation, protect joint health, and support your body as it moves through each decade. With regular practice, you'll feel more energized, more stable, and more connected to your physical strength.

SLOW, STEADY MOVEMENT FOR SUSTAINABLE RESULTS

Unlike fast-paced, high-intensity programs, chair yoga is based on slow, controlled movements that are deeply effective. Each stretch and posture is designed to be fully felt—so you get more out of less. You don't need to sweat buckets to make progress. You just need to show up, breathe deeply, and move with care.

Over time, you'll likely notice improvements not only in your body but in your mindset. You may feel less anxious, more confident, and more in tune with your needs. That's the beauty of this practice—it transforms from the inside out.

A COMPASSIONATE PRACTICE WITHOUT COMPETITION

There's no room for comparison here. You're not racing anyone. You don't need to be perfect or push through pain. This practice is about honoring your body, listening to your limits, and building trust in yourself.

Chair yoga encourages a non-competitive, judgment-free environment where every movement is a celebration of what your body can do. Whether you're lifting a leg, holding a stretch, or simply breathing mindfully—you are doing the work. And that is enough.

READY TO BEGIN?

Take a few deep breaths, find a comfortable chair, and open your heart to this new journey. You deserve to feel good in your body. You deserve to move with confidence, strength, and joy. This book is here to support you every step of the way.

Let's begin—together.

HOW TO DOWNLOAD YOUR BONUS

ACCESS VIDEOS AND OTHER BONUS CONTENT:

Thank you so much for choosing this book. I created it with the hope that it would feel like a supportive companion; something simple, uplifting, and truly approachable as you begin your journey.

To get started, I recommend following the daily plan outlined at the back of your book. Each chart is a gentle guide for one day of movement. You're welcome to complete it once a day or repeat it if you're feeling energized. In the early days, take things slow and notice how your body feels with each exercise. As your confidence grows, you might choose to repeat the routine two or three times in a row, with a 3-minute pause between each round. There's no rush—listen to your body and honor your pace with kindness.

And don't forget—the videos are here to support you every step of the way. I included one for each exercise so you can clearly see how the movements flow, reducing any guesswork and helping you stay safe. You can access them anytime from your phone, tablet, or computer, whenever it's most convenient for you. It's all about making this journey feel smooth, empowering, and uniquely yours.

ARE YOU READY?

LET'S GO!

1 SPINAL TWIST

This movement will be able to stretch the abdominal muscles and the spine. It will help you relax and erase all the possible tension accumulated in your day. You will feel an elongation on the entire back, especially on the lower part.

Step by Step Instructions

1. Sit on the chair, keep your spine straight, by endorsing your back and shoulders on your backrest
2. Twist to your right side, place your right hand on your backrest and your left had on the seat.
3. Hold on this position for 5 seconds and then come back to the starting position
4. Conduct the same movement to your left side

Tips and Tricks

During the execution of this exercise, I recommend you keep your feet on the floor with your legs straight. Focus only on the twisting movement. If you are still learning, do not strain your back too much because you can conduct a partial twist. Over time you will start to execute the movement without issues.

Breathing

Exhale when you are twisting and inhale when you are coming back to the initial position.

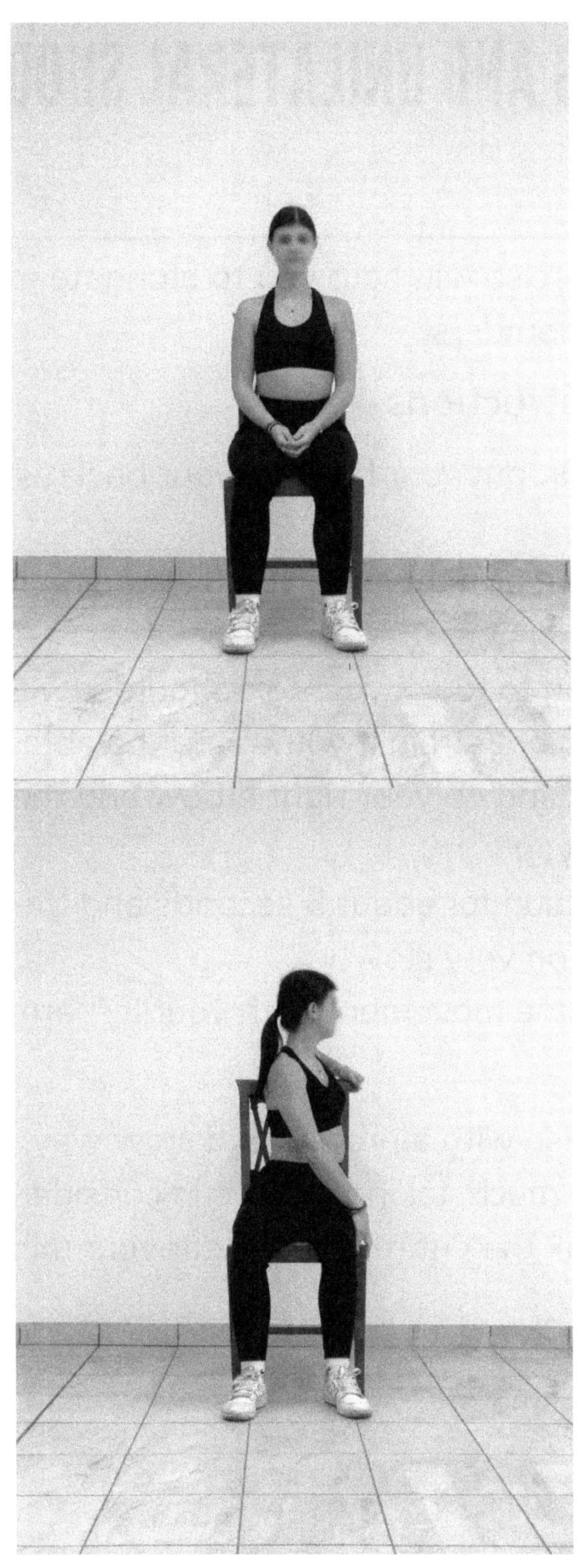

2 STRETCHING AND UNILATERAL SHOULDERS ELONGATION

This stretching exercise will help you to elongate muscles along the backside of your shoulders.

Step by Step Instructions

1. Sit on the chair, put your back on your backrest and your feet on the floor
2. Bring your right arm towards you by keeping it as tense as you can
3. Imagine having to touch your left shoulder with your right arm (be careful, do not strain if you cannot be able to do it)
4. Put your left hand on your right elbow and then push your right arm towards you
5. Hold this position for about 5 seconds and then return to the starting position very slowly
6. Repeat the same movement with your left arm

Tips and Tricks

Conduct this exercise with a precise and slow way, without straining your shoulders too much, taking always in consideration that the main goal is to relax the entire body. Clear your mind and focus entirely on you.

Breathing

Breathe normally.

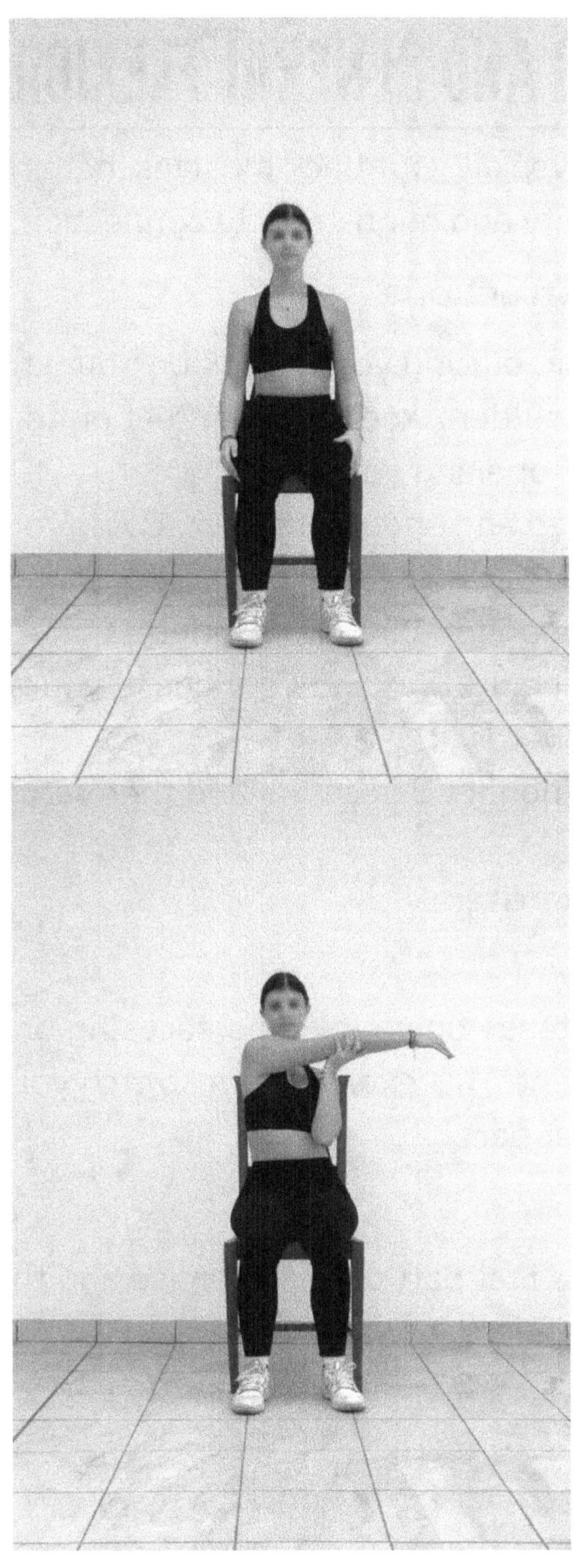

3 STRETCHING AND GENERAL FLEXIBILITY

This exercise involves all your back muscles, helping you to improve the general flexibility and mind-muscle connection.

Step by Step Instructions

1. Sit on the chair, placing your hands on your knees
2. Relax your shoulders, keeping your feet on the floor
3. Inhale deeply, opening your chest
4. Bring your head and shoulders back, trying to get your shoulder blades close
5. Hold this position for about 3 seconds
6. Now exhale deeply, bringing your chest, your head, and your shoulders forward
7. Hold this position for 3 seconds and then return to the starting position
8. Repeat the exercise

Tips and Tricks

Keep your hands steady on your knees, focusing only on your shoulder's movement. This exercise can stretch your entire back, especially the upper part.

Breathing

Inhale deeply in the first part of this exercise and then exhale with you bring your shoulders forward.

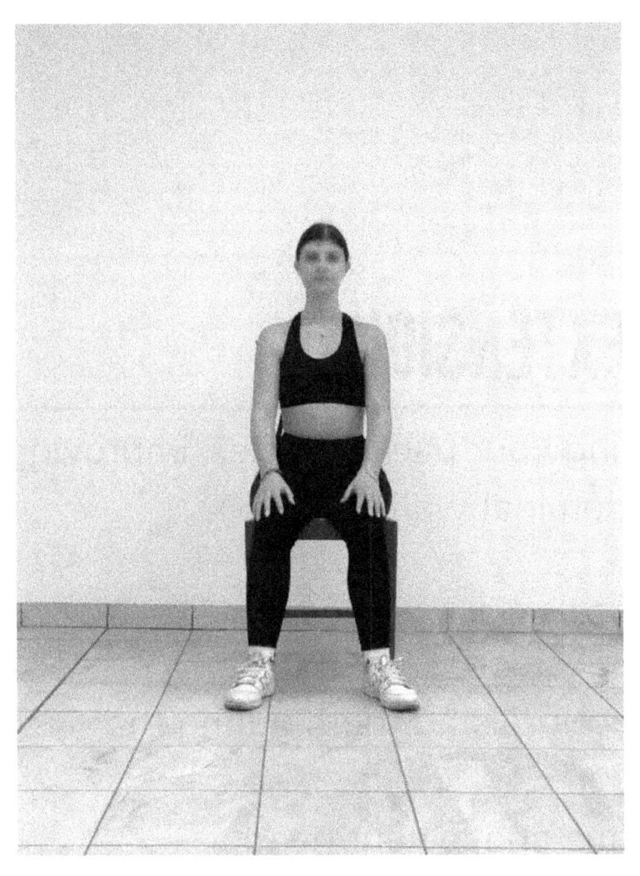
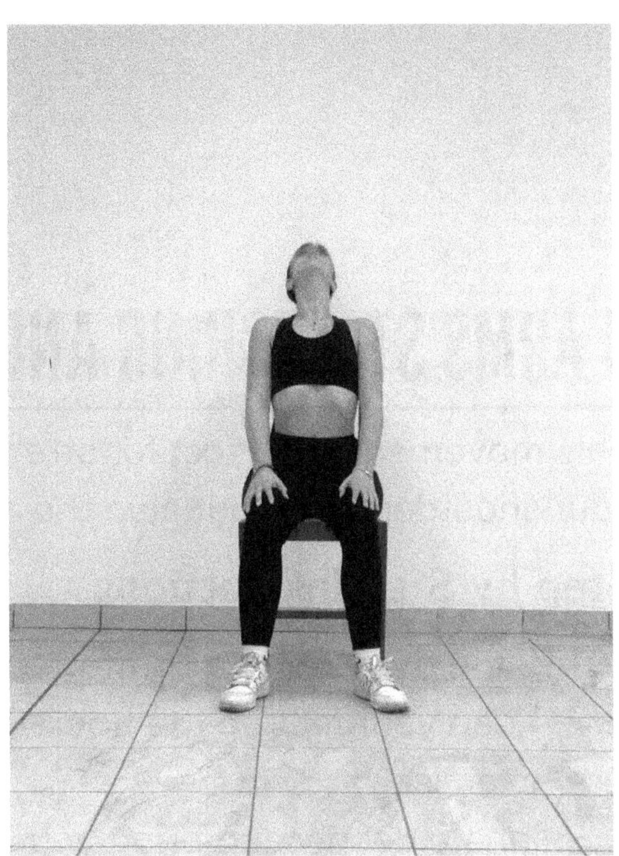
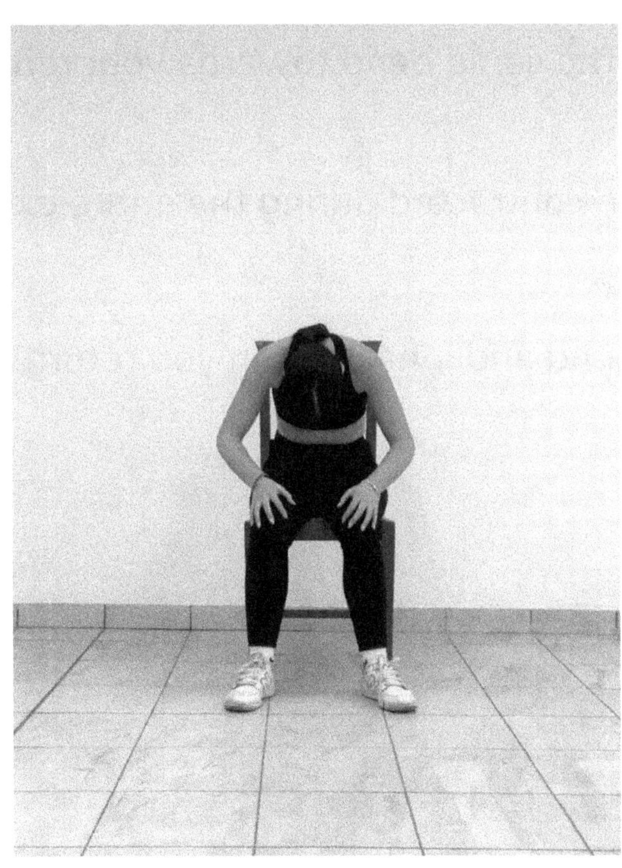

4 ARMS STRETCHING AND EXTENSION

This movement is perfect for stretching your back muscles, improving your shoulders back but also the abdominal wall.

Step by Step Instructions

1. Sit in the chair in a comfortable position
2. Keep your feet on the floor without raising them during the exercise.
3. Inhale deeply and bring your arms above your head
4. Put your hands together and bend towards your right side
5. Now perform the same bend towards your left side

Tips and Tricks

Keep your abdomen contracted during the entire exercise without

Breathing

Exhale when you bend and inhale when you return to the starting position

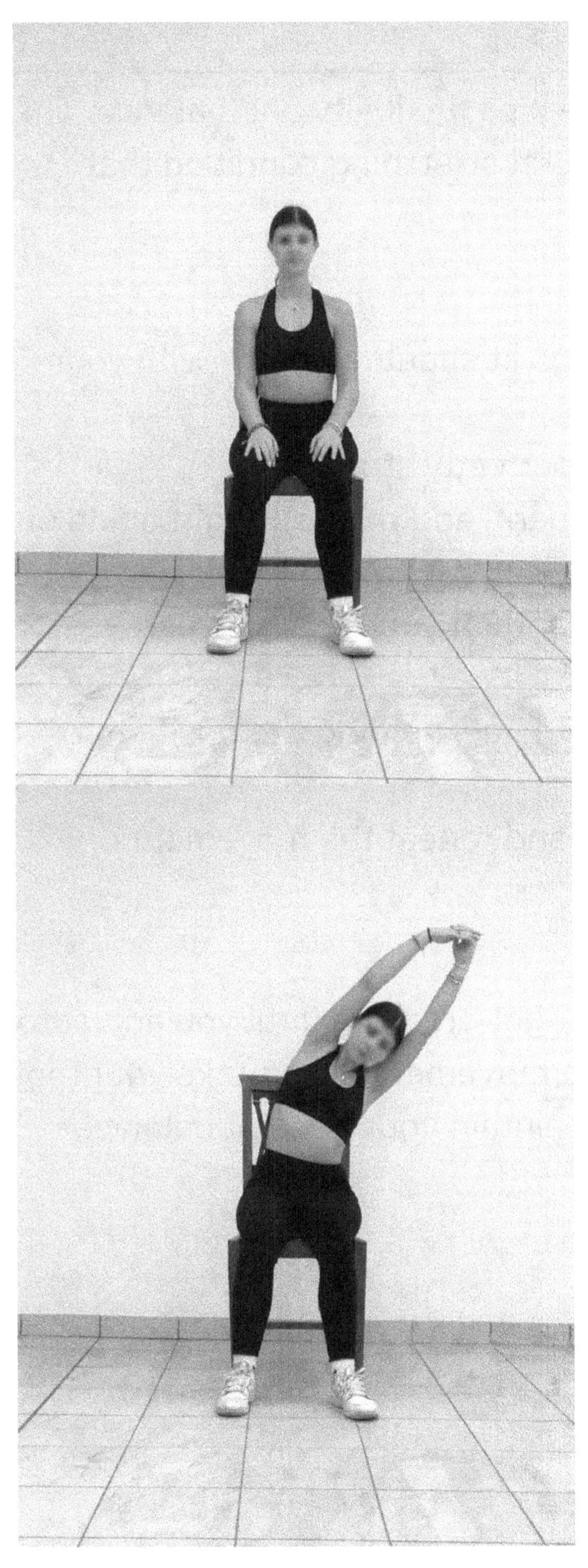
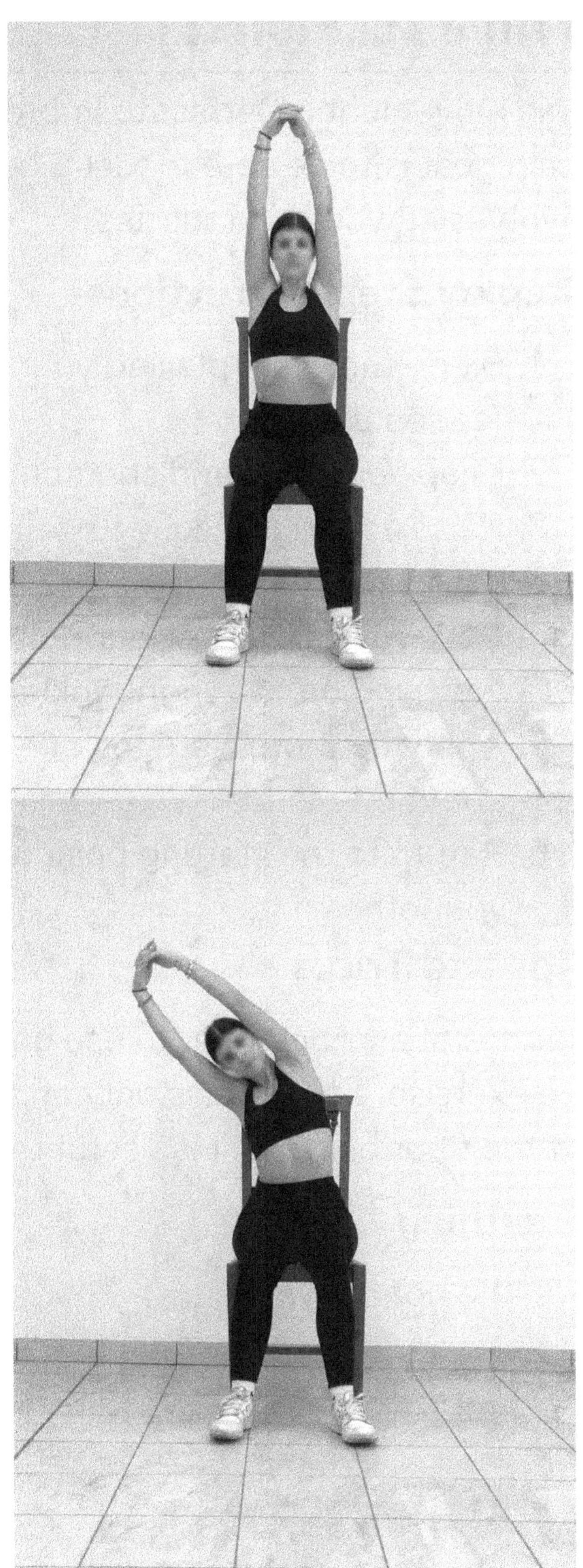

5 HIPS FLEXIBILITY

This movement is perfect to improve hips flexibility and balance. The main goal is to be able to feel a general stretching condition that involves all your leg muscles.

Step by Step Instructions

1. Sit on the chair, placing your legs at shoulder width with your feet on the floor.
2. Keep your back and shoulders perfectly straight
3. Raise your right leg, with knee bent, and put your right ankle on your left knee
4. Now you can place your right hand on your left knee and your left hand on your right ankle
5. Apply light pressure to your left knee, holding the position for about 5 seconds
6. Return to the starting position, and repeat the movement on your other side

Tips and Tricks

Be careful as a beginner to use only light pressure until you adjust to the exercise. Try to focus only on the movement. Don't take your foot off the floor because it is useful to maintain your general balance.

Breathing

Breathe normally.

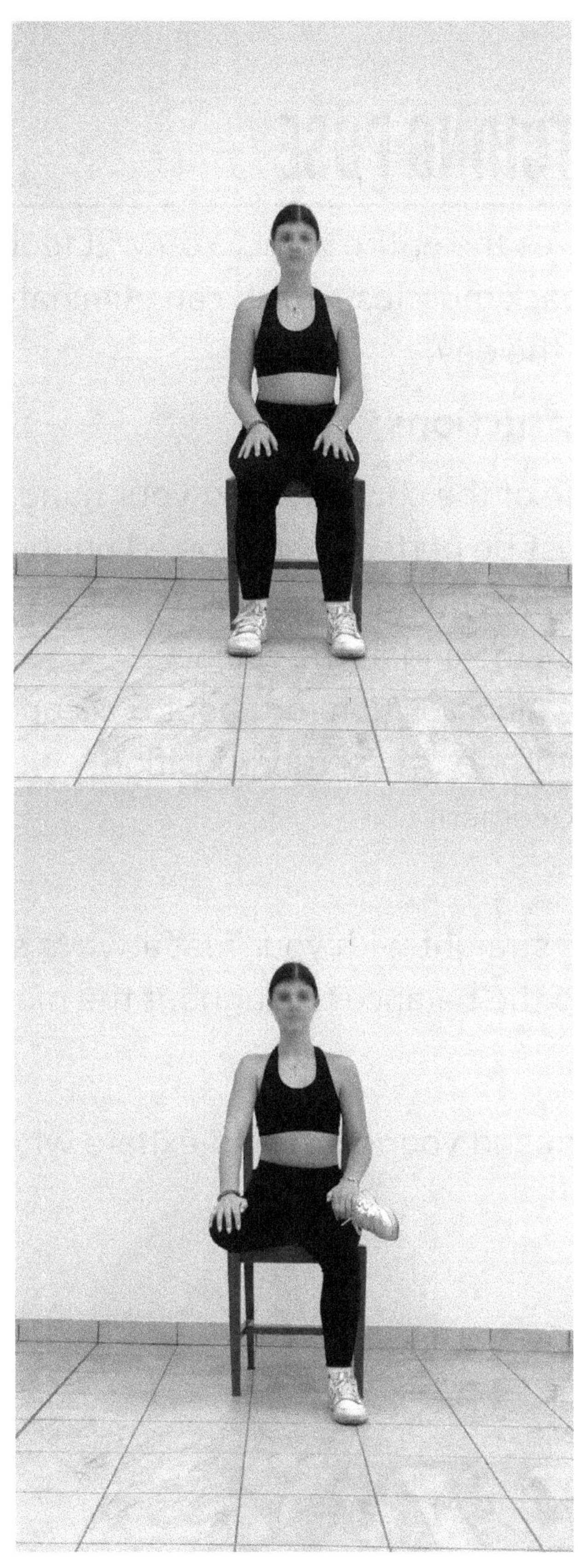

6 SPINE STRETCHING POSE

This exercise involves the entire spine. You will feel a general activation of your back muscles, which can eliminate tension you can accumulate during the day.

Step by Step Instructions

1. Sit on the edge of the chair, placing your hands near your hips
2. The glutes must be perfectly supported on the chair
3. Inhale deeply, expanding your chest
4. Raise your chin, looking at the ceiling
5. Hold the stretching position for about 5 seconds
6. Exhale and return to the starting position
7. Repeat the movement

Tips and Tricks

Maintain your arms straight with your feet always on the floor. You will be able to keep the balance throughout the movement.

Breathing

Inhale when you expand your chest and exhale when you return to the starting position.

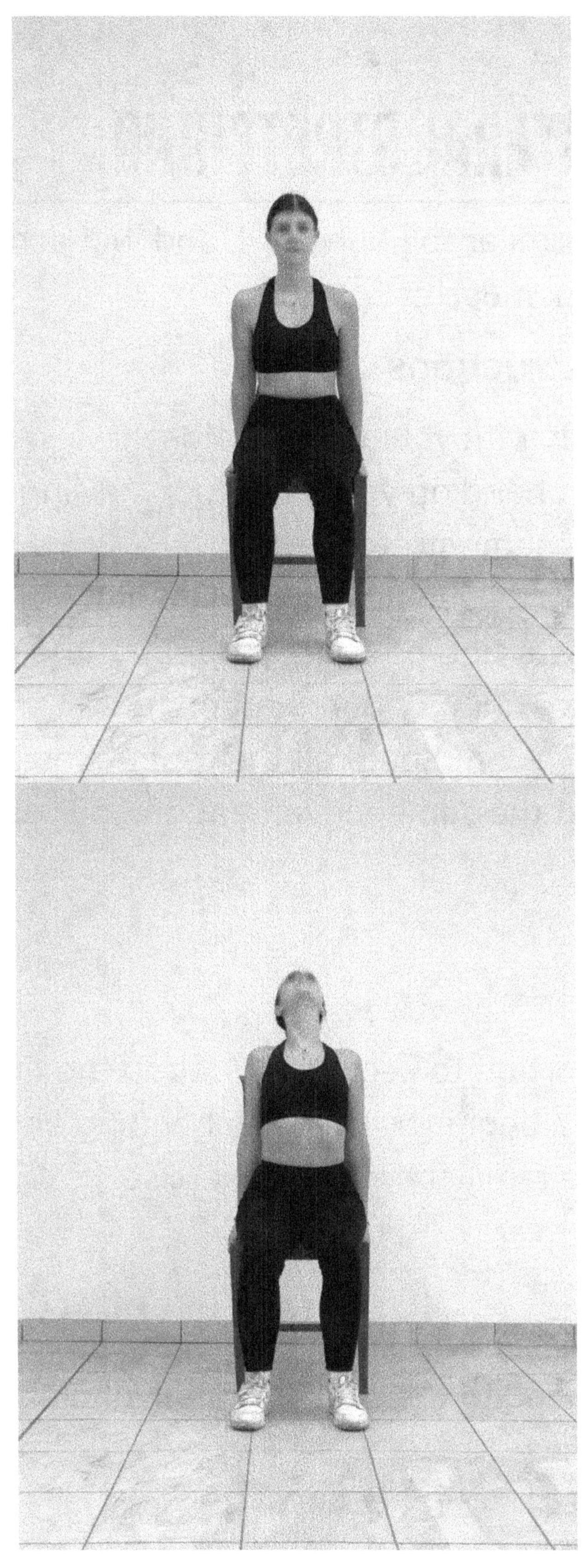

7 ARMS UNILATERAL STRETCHING

This movement is similar to Exercise 4, and will activate all your abdominal and back muscles.

Step by Step Instructions

1. Sit on the chair with your back straight
2. Place your left hand on your abdomen, raising your right arm and keeping it semi-stretched
3. Bend to your left, keeping focus on your abdomen
4. Return to the starting position and repeat the movement (see the program for number of repetitions)
5. When you have completed all the repetitions on your left side, you can repeat the same movement on your right with your left arm raised

Tips and Tricks

It is extremely important to keep your feet on the floor to maintain balance. If you are a beginner, keep the bending and stretching gentle until you are familiar with the exercise.

Breathing

Exhale when you bend to the side and then inhale when you return to the starting position.

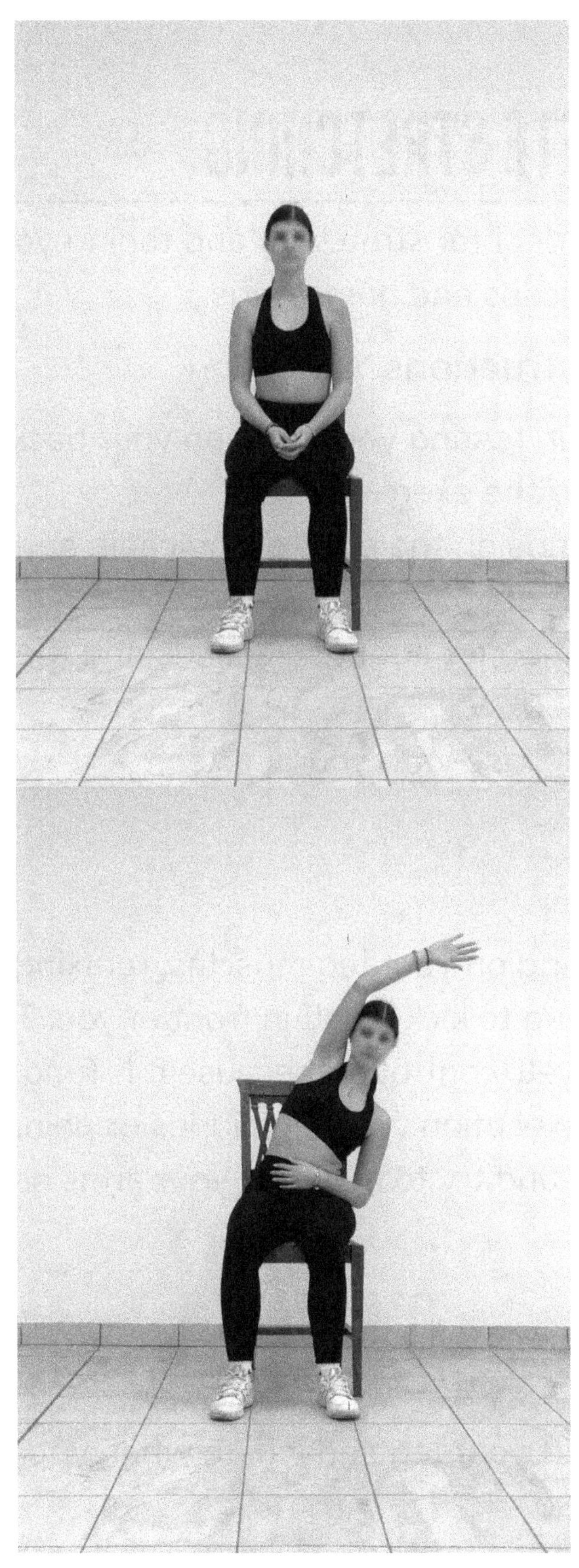

8 LEG COMPLETE STRETCHING

This movement is ideal for stretching and toning your leg muscles. It involves the quadriceps and hamstrings.

Step by Step Instructions

1. Sit on the chair, resting your back on your backrest to maintain it straight during the exercise
2. Place your hands on the edge of the chair, and extend your right leg out in front of you
3. Hold this position for about 5 seconds and then return to the starting position
4. Repeat the exercise with your left leg

Tips and Tricks

The secret is focusing on your leg muscles, relaxing the rest of the body. Imagine having to kick a ball in front of you. The movement must be soft and well-controlled because it is fundamental to conduct a correct execution without injuries or pain. Never take your hands off the chair and try to maintain your arms as straight as you can.

Breathing

Exhale when you lift your leg and inhale when you return to the starting position.

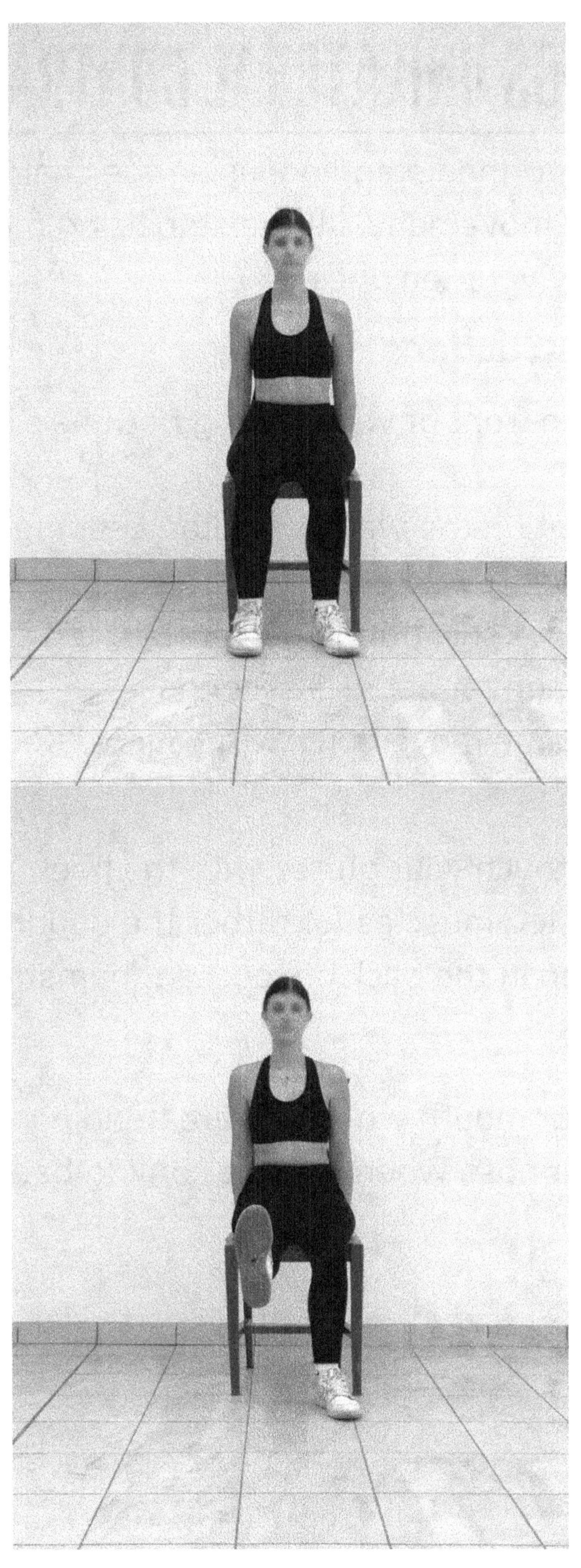

9 HARMSTRINGS UNILATERAL CONTRACTION

This exercise is performed standing, using the chair to maintain balance during the movement. All the stabilizing muscles will be involved, especially your leg ones.

Step by Step Instructions

1. Put the chair in front of you, placing both hands on the back of the chair
2. Stare at a point on the wall or similar, keeping your focus only on the movement
3. Bend your right knee, bringing your right leg backwards, and hold this position for about 5 seconds
4. Perform the same movement with your left leg

Tips and Tricks

Imagine having to touch your glutes with the heel. You will feel a stretch in the front leg muscles (or rather the quadriceps) and a stronger contraction in the back of your leg (hamstrings).

Breathing

Exhale through your mouth when you are bending your knee, then inhale through your nose when you are coming back to the initial position.

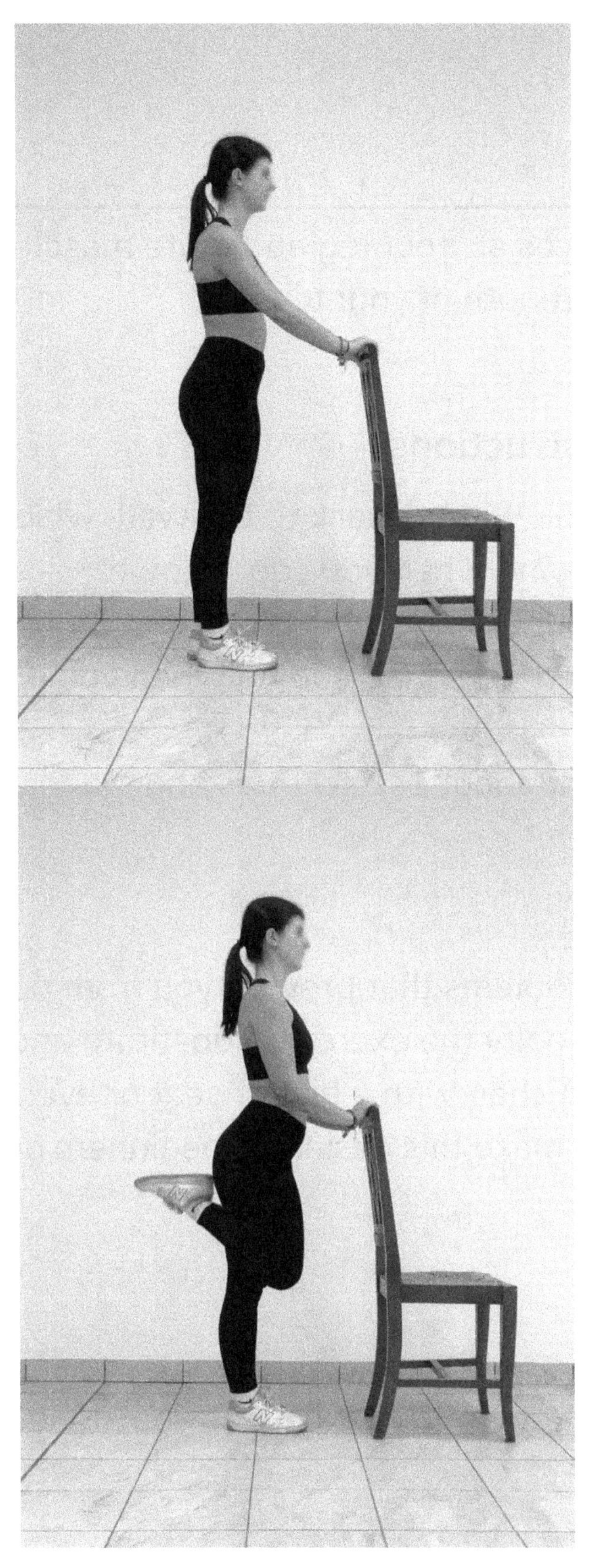

10 SQUATS

This exercise involves all your leg and glute muscles, improving balance and the strength of your legs.

Step by Step Instructions

1. Place your chair with its back to the wall, which will keep the chair from moving when you squat down
2. Stand with your arms extended at shoulder height
3. Bend your knees to squat, ending when you are sitting on the chair
4. Stay seated for about 1-2 seconds and stand up

Tips and Tricks

If you have knee problems that prevent you from performing this full exercise you can modify the exercise, substitute another one, or even skip it altogether. A chair with a higher seat or even with a pillow on top of the seat can make this easier for beginners or those with knee challenges.

Breathing

Inhale as you squat down, and exhale as you stand back up.

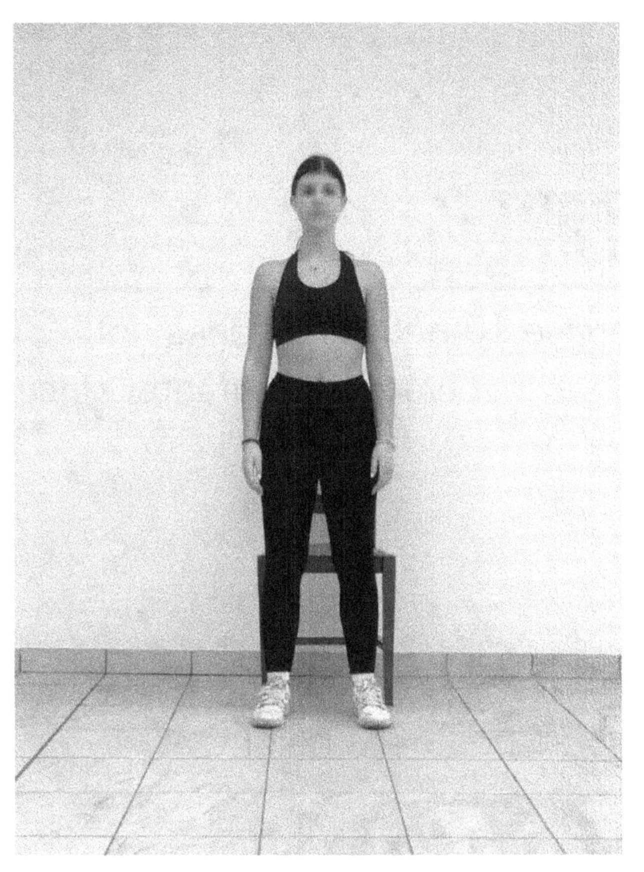 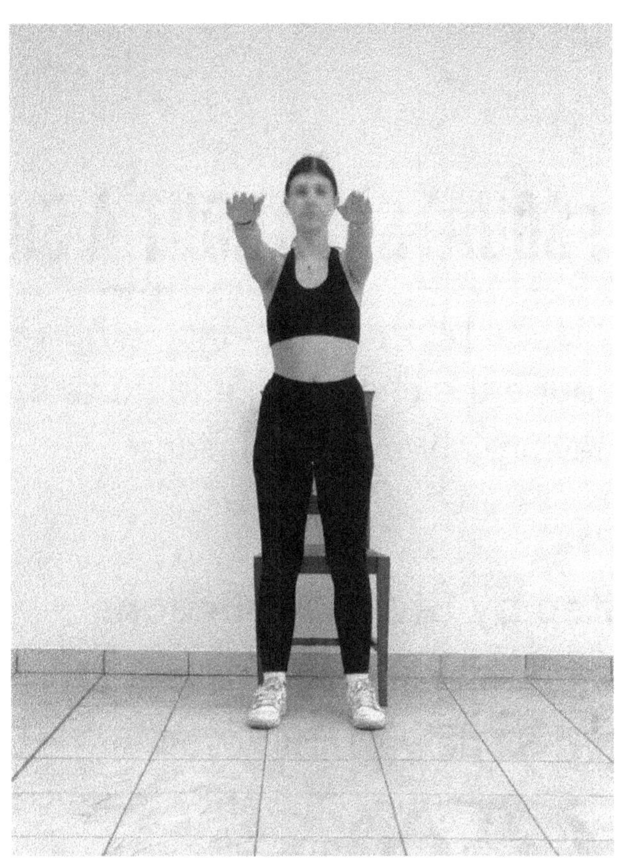

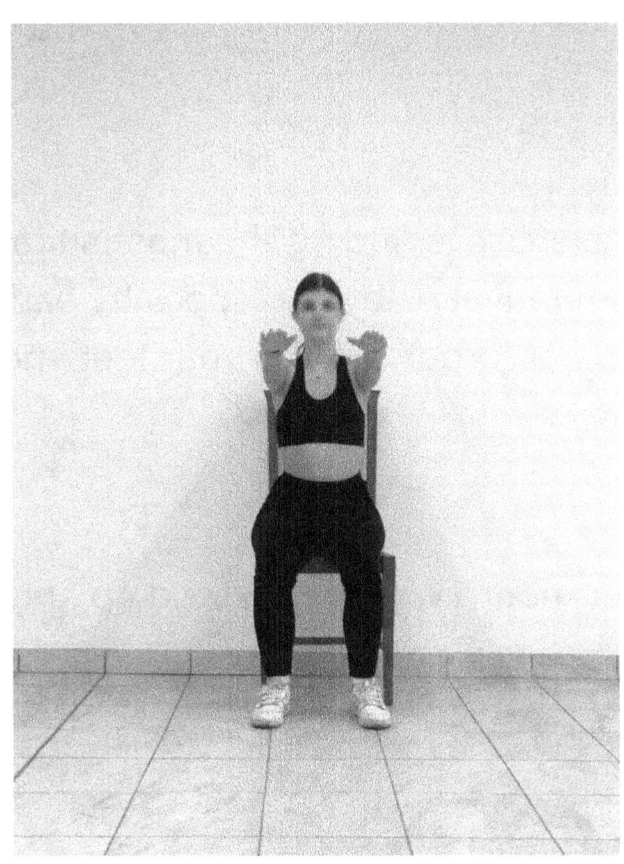

11 SQUATS WITHOUT A SUPPORT

This is a bit more advanced than Exercise 10 because it does not require the chair. Leg and glute muscles involvement is greater since they are always in tension.

Step by Step Instructions

1. Stand in front of the chair
2. Sit down, raising your arms to your shoulder's height, always keeping them well-straight
3. Squat until you can touch the chair
4. Return to the starting position without sitting on the chair

Tips and Tricks

The secret for this exercise is finding the most suitable place for you. Make sure to move relatively slowly, especially early on as you learn the proper form. Do not forget to keep your feet shoulder width.

Breathing

Exhale through your mouth when you stand up and inhale when you bend down.

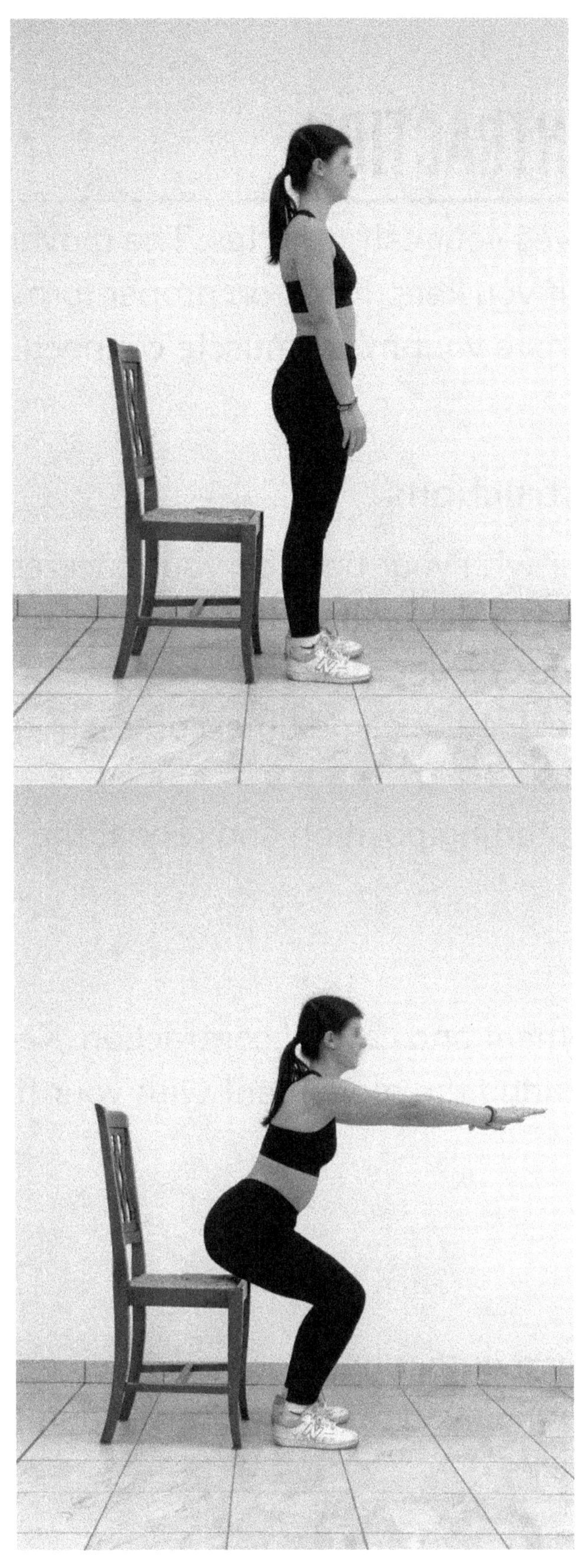

12 CALVES CONTRACTION

This exercise involves your calf muscles. The movement appears very simple at first, but if you keep focus on proper form every time, you will be able to improve your mind-muscle connection.

Step by Step Instructions

1. Sit on the chair with your back on your backrest
2. Keep your feet parallel and well-supported on the floor
3. Place your hands on your knees
4. Raise both heels at the same time, contracting your calves for about 5 seconds
5. Return to the starting position and repeat the same movement

Tips and Tricks

Focus on the movement and calves' contraction. Keep your back perfectly straight during the movement with your hands on your knees.

Breathing

Exhale through your mouth when you raise the heels and then, inhale through your nose when you return to the starting position

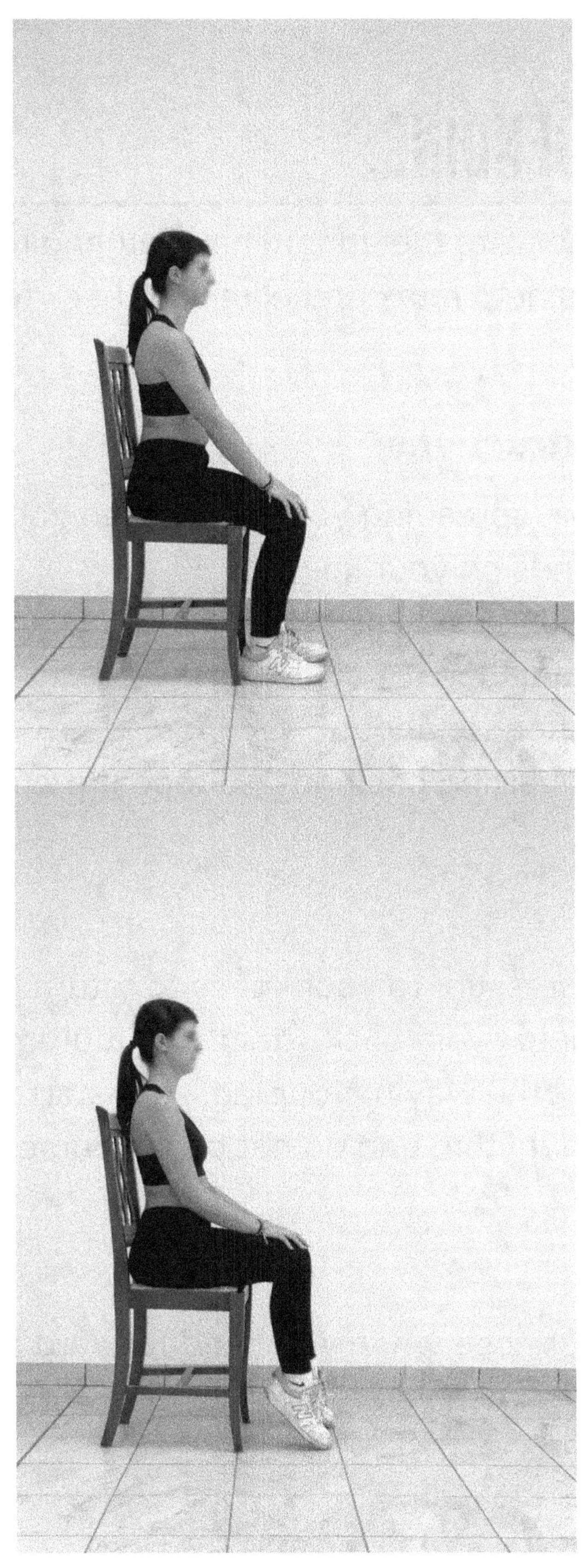

13 FORWARD BENDING

This exercise can activate the abdominal wall and lower back muscles. It can also help relax and eliminate back tension.

Step by Step Instructions

1. Sit on the chair, spreading your wider than your shoulders
2. Place your hands on your knees
3. Bend forward as far as you comfortably can, staring at a fixed point flat on the floor
4. Hold this position for about 5 seconds
5. Return to the starting position and repeat the same exercise

Tips and Tricks

Apply some hand pressure to your knees to return to the starting position; this will help avoid back strain. You'll ultimately want to try to get your chest all the way to your legs, but start slowly and work p to it. Find your own rhythm and do not push yourself especially if you are a beginner.

Breathing

Exhale through your nose when you bend forward and inhale through your mouth when you return to the starting position.

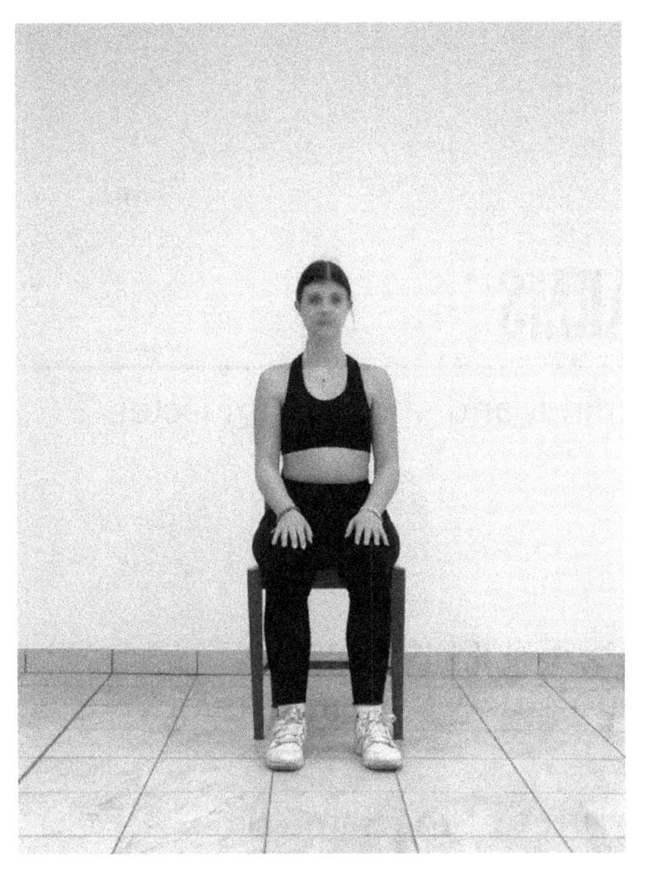

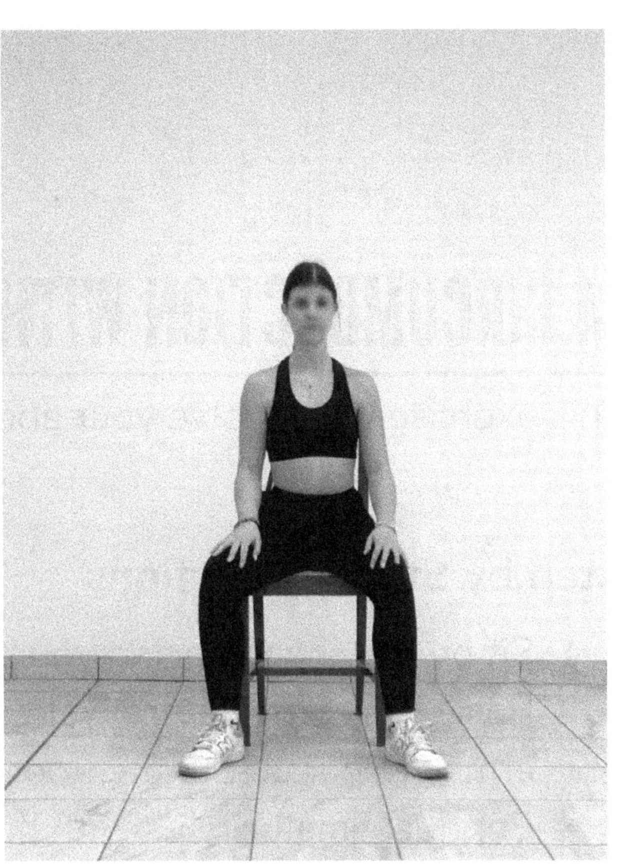

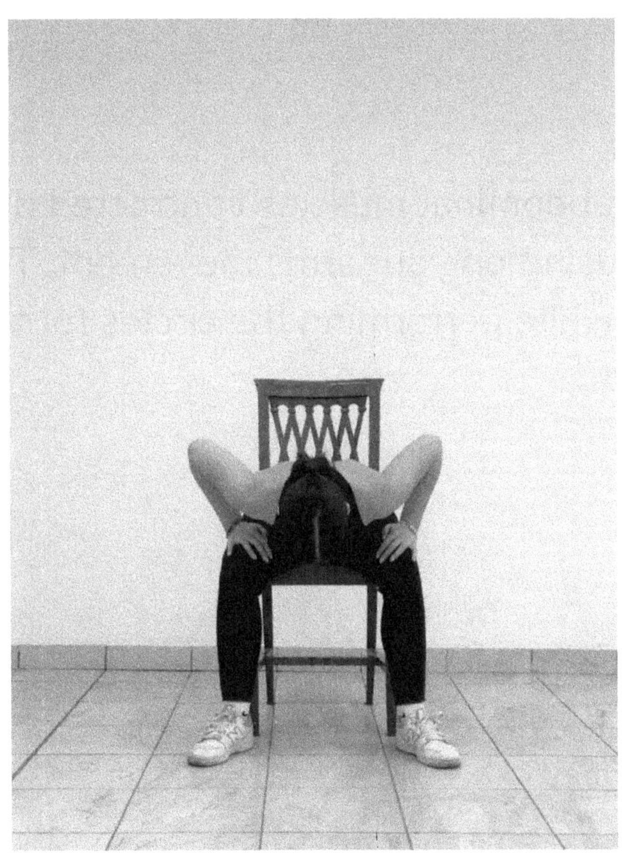

14 CIRCUMDUCTION WITH ARMS

This exercise will involve your abdominal and shoulder muscles.

Step by Step Instructions

1. Sit on the chair, placing your legs at shoulder width
2. Raise your arms laterally, keeping elbows straight, until your arms are parallel to the floor
3. Conduct small circles with both arms at the same time
4. Follow the instructions present in the training program

Tips and Tricks

Always keep your abdominal muscles contracted during the entire exercise, while focusing on your arms movement. Try to keep your shoulders relaxed while performing the circles for the most benefit.

Breathing

Breathe normally.

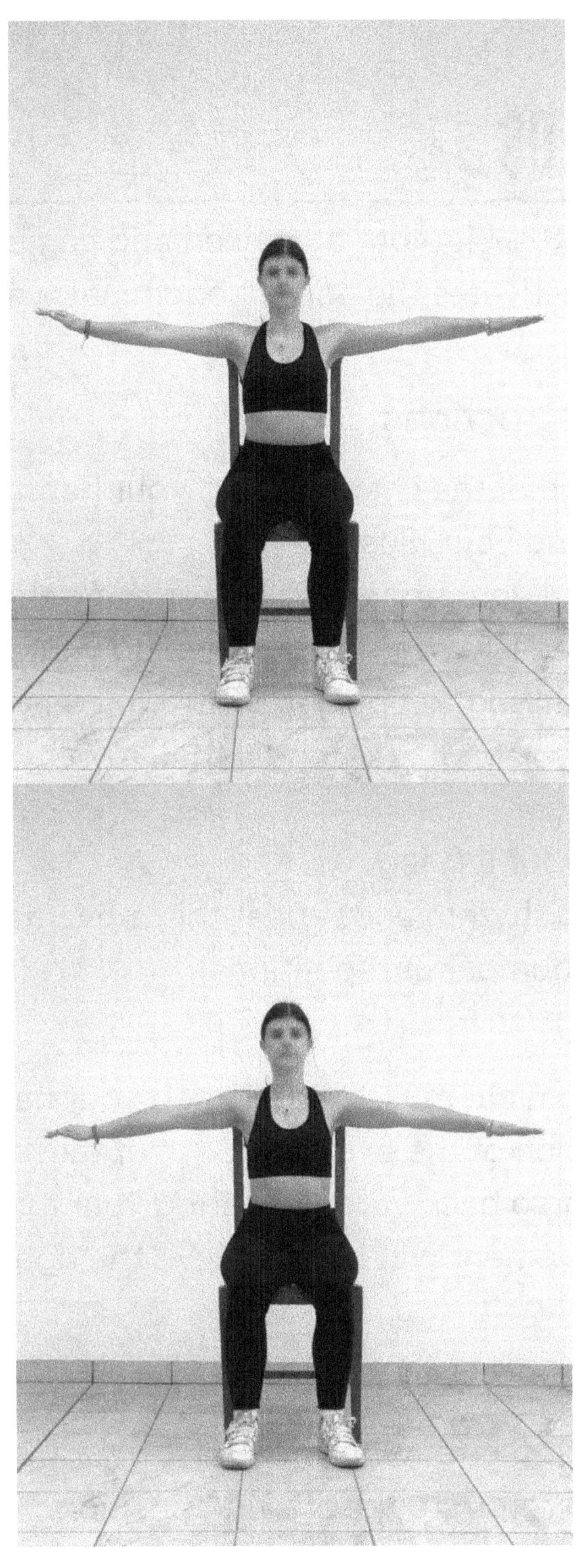

15 SCISSOR LEGS

This exercise is a little bit more advanced and complicated than the others because it activates the entire abdominal wall and leg muscles.

Step by Step Instructions

1. Sit on the edge of the chair, placing your hands on the side of the chair behind your hips
2. Lean back until your upper back is touching the back of the chair
3. Extend your legs in front of you, keeping your heels on the floor
4. Raise your right leg, keeping it as straight as you can, and hold this position for about 3 seconds, then lower until your heel touches the floor
5. Repeat with your left leg
6. Find your own rhythm and repeat this movement (daily video program has number of repetitions)

Tips and Tricks

Contract your abdominal muscles and keep your hands on the chair for the entire duration of the exercise. Both of these will help stabilize as you lean your torso backwards. Clearing your mind and thinking only about the movement will help achieve the right form for the exercise.

Breathing

Exhale through your mouth when you raise your leg and inhale with the nose when you return to the starting position.

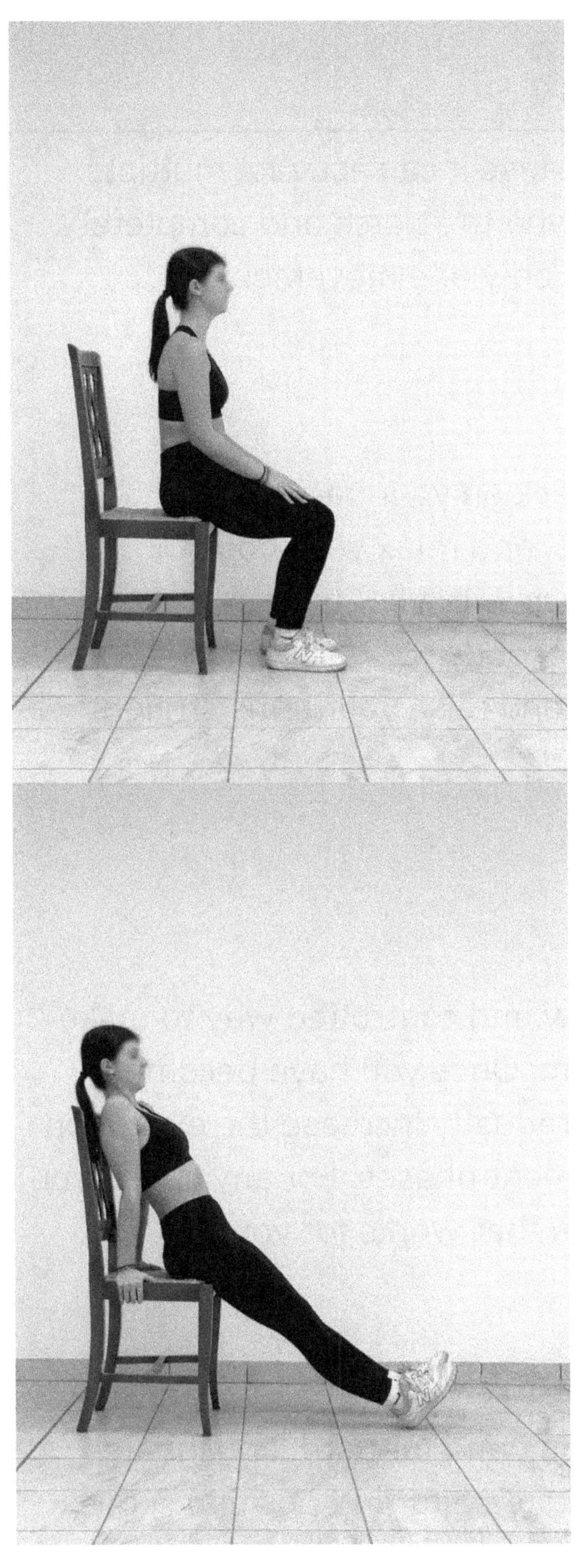
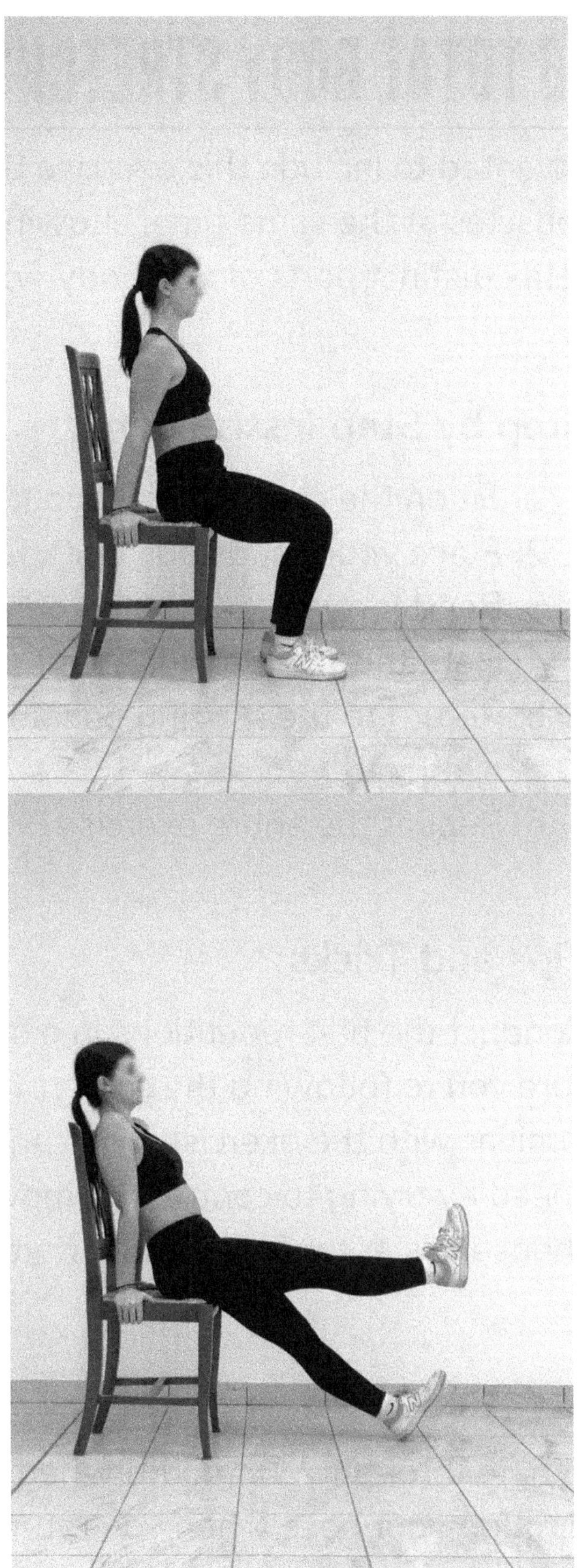

16 TOTAL BODY STRETCHING

I wanted to include this exercise because it can activate multiple muscles at the same time, allowing you to stretch and completely relax distinct parts of you body with only one movement.

Step by Step Instructions

1. Sit on the chair and rest your back on your backrest
2. Place your hands on your knees, and relax your body
3. Bend forward, touching your toes with your hands
4. Hold this position for about 5 seconds
5. Return to the starting position, and raise your arms straight overhead
6. Repeat the entire exercise

Tips and Tricks

Conduct the first repetitions in a slow and controlled way to make sure you're following the correct form. Once you have become familiar with the exercise, you can gradually increase the execution speed by trying to control the movement phases. For any speed you choose, it's essential to find a rhythm that works for you.

Breathing

Exhale through your mouth when you bend forward, and inhale through your nose when you return to the starting position & raise your arms.

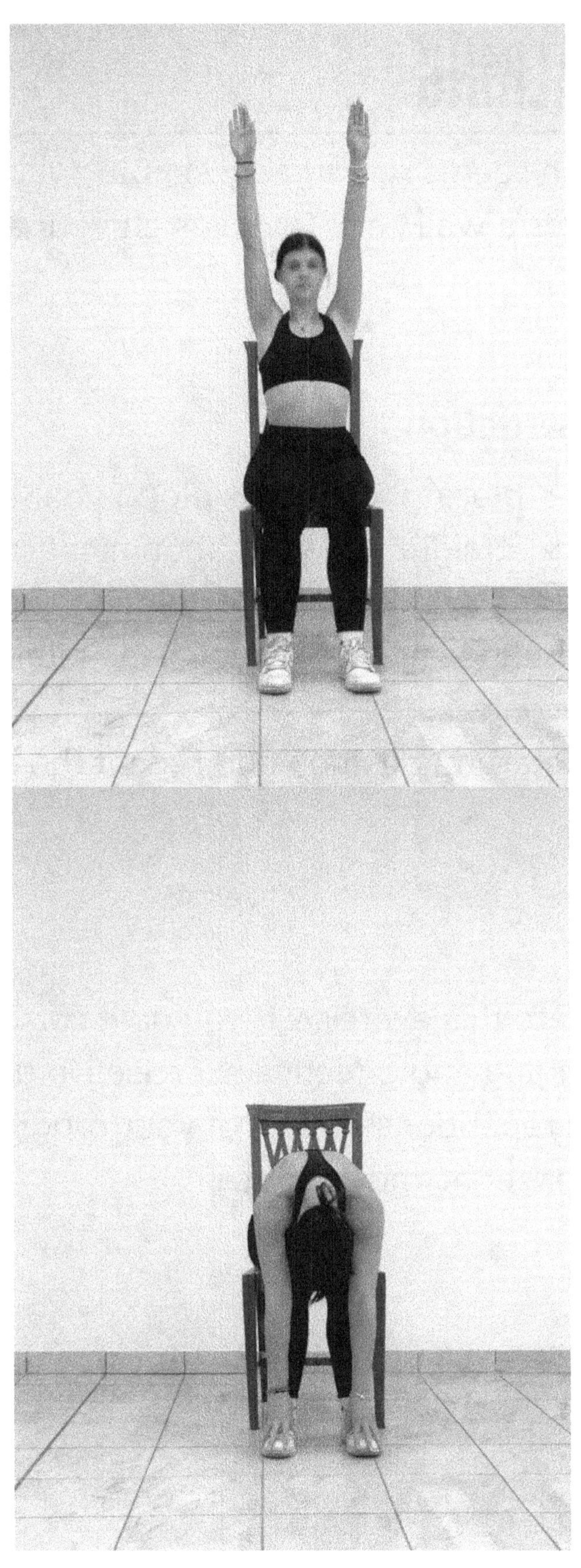

17 SEATED WALKING

This exercise, which seems remarkably simple, will surprise you! The movement simulates a walk, and involves all your abdominal and legs muscles.

Step by Step Instructions

1. Sit on the chair, placing your arms along your sides
2. Keep your back straight and your abdominal muscles contracted
3. Raise your right leg as if you were going to take a step
4. Bring your right knee as high as you can, holding this position for about 3 seconds
5. Return to the starting position and repeat the exercise with your left leg

Tips and Tricks

Do not underestimate this exercise: if you do it correctly, it can be one of the most challenging and effective exercises in this book. Try it 2-3 times before doing repetitions as part of your program to understand and begin to memorize the movement.

Breathing

Inhale when you raise your knee and exhale when you lower it.

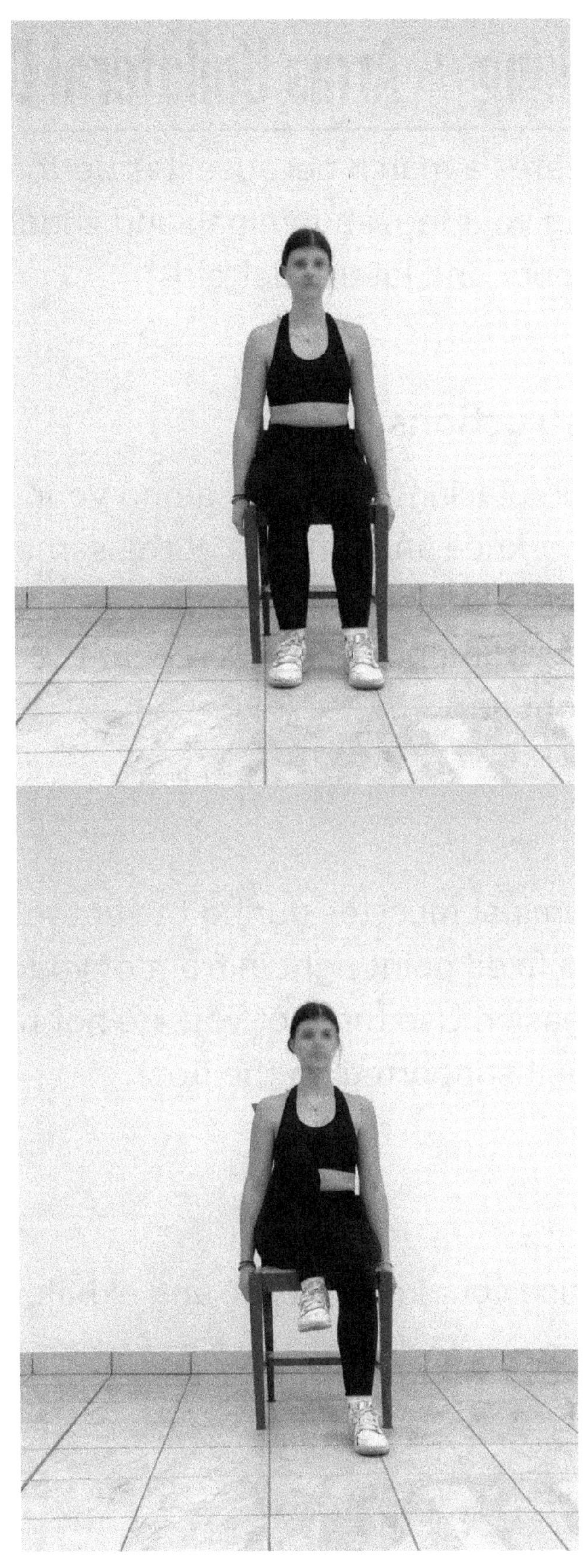

18 Seated Walking + Arms Unilateral Distension

This exercise simulates a march because it is performed while you are sitting, involving your leg, abdominal, and shoulder muscles (primarily your anterior and lateral deltoids).

Step by Step Instructions

1. Sit on the chair, placing your arms along your sides
2. Raise your right knee and left arm at the same time
3. Hold this position for about 3 seconds
4. Return to the starting position and repeat the exercise with your left leg and right arm

Tips and Tricks

Contract your abdominal muscles during the entire exercise. It's helpful to stare at a fixed point right in front of you to make focusing on the movement easier. Use the foot you are not raising to help you keep balanced & well supported on the floor.

Breathing

Inhale when you raise your knee & arm, and exhale when you lower them.

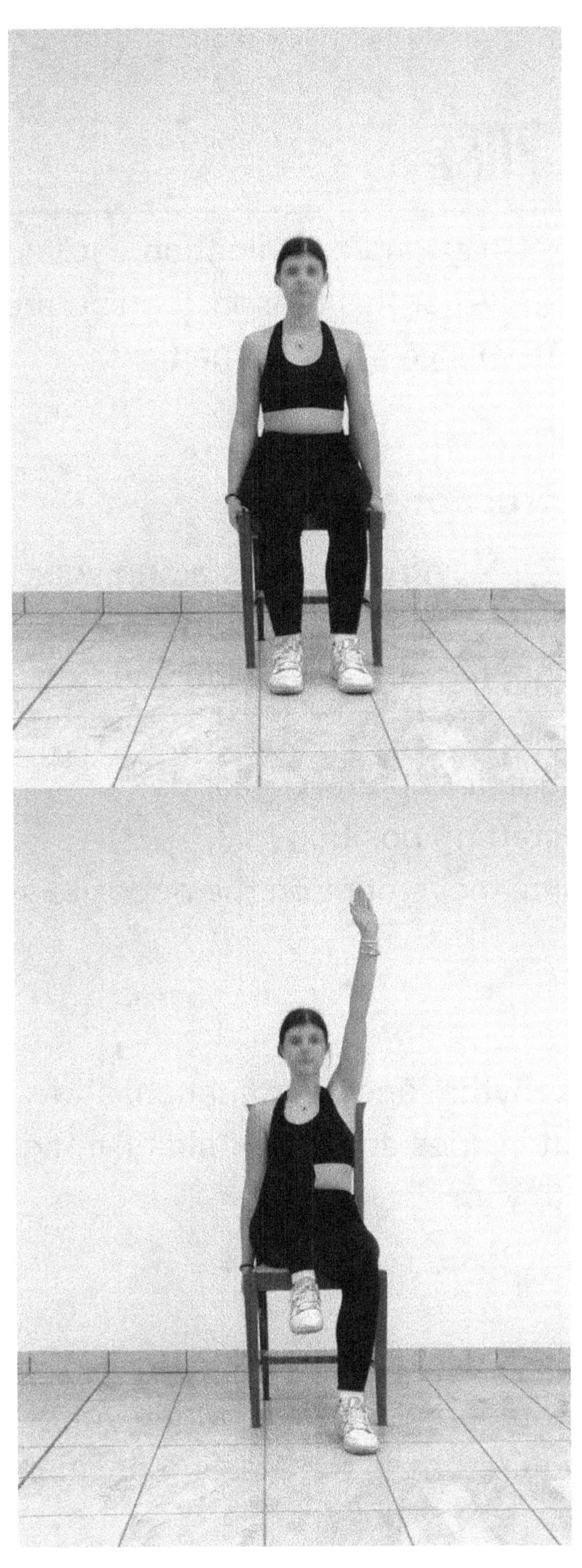

19 SUPERMAN POSE

This exercise requires a strong coordination between the upper and lower parts of the body. For this reason, leg and arm muscles will be involved in this performance at the same time.

Step by Step Instructions

1. Sit on the chair, placing your arms along your sides
2. Place your feet shoulder width apart
3. Spread your right leg out, extending your left arm to your right with a pelvis rotation
4. Hold this position for about 3 seconds
5. Return to the starting position
6. Repeat the same movement on the opposite side

Tips and Tricks

Focus on your right rhythm and coordination, allowing you to conduct the exercise without injuries and with fluidity. Imagine having to push something hard with your fist.

Breathing

Exhale through your mouth when you widen your leg and extend the arm. Inhale when you return to the starting position.

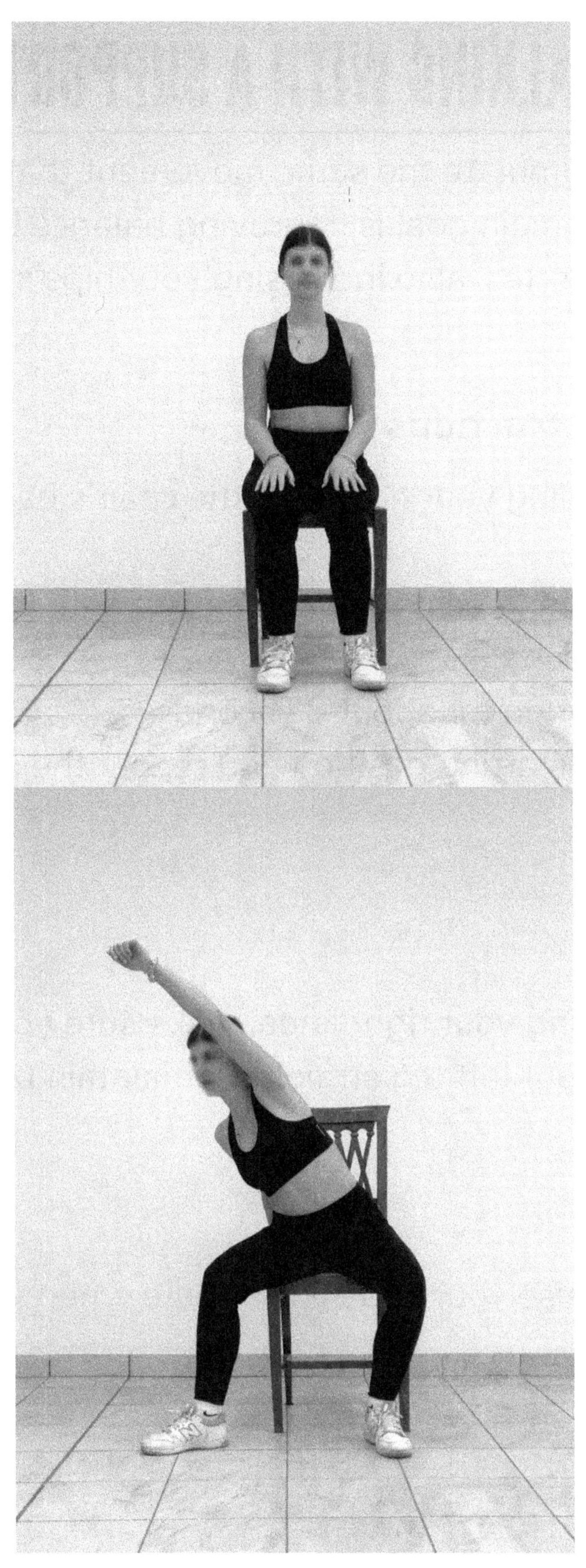

20 SEATED WALKING WITH A SUPPORT

This exercise can simulate the same movement that we do daily during a walk. The main goal is improving balance by improving leg and abdominal muscles, also increasing your hips' mobility.

Step by Step Instructions

1. Stand up, placing your hands on the chair's back with your arms outstretched
2. Raise your right knee until it's at a 90° angle (or as close as you can get)
3. Hold this position for about 3 seconds
4. Return to the starting position and repeat the movement with your left leg

Tips and Tricks

When you are raising your right knee, make sure your left foot is flat on the floor with your left leg straight to maintain balance.

Breathing

Inhale when you raise your knee and exhale when you lower it.

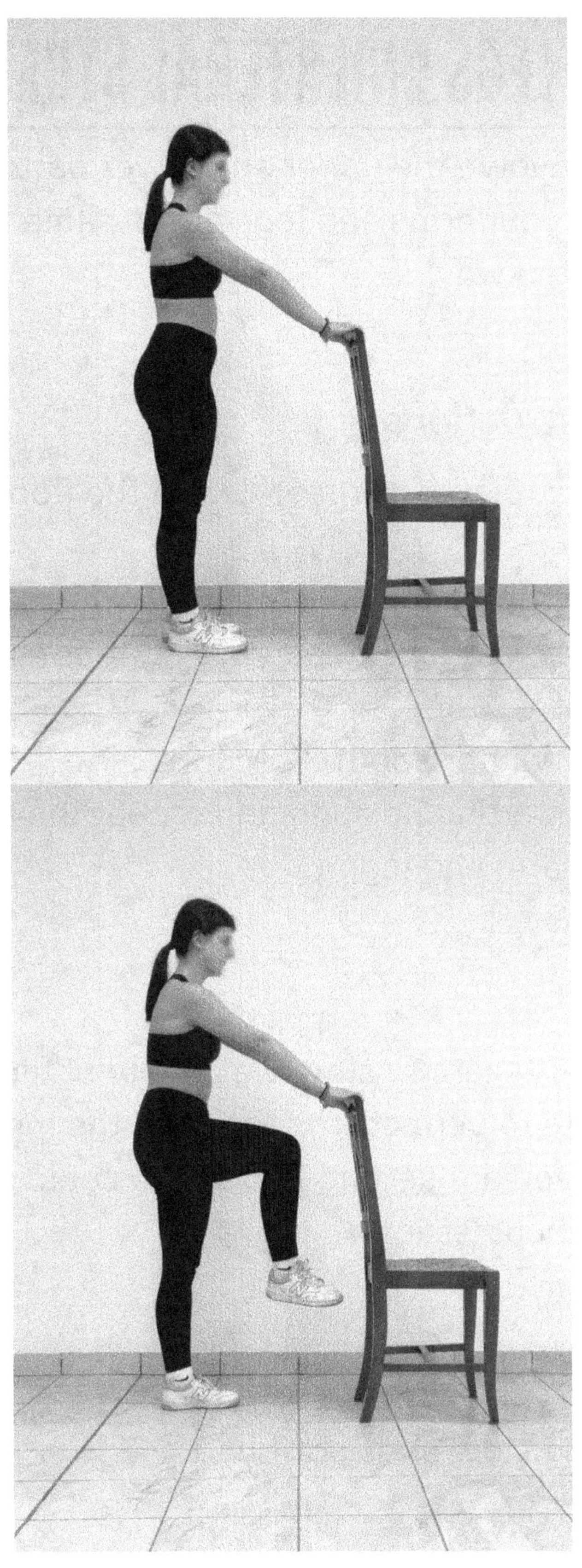

21 ARMS AND LEGS UNILATERAL STRETCHING

This exercise will involve the upper and lower parts of the body, having you extend your arms and legs at the same time in a unilateral and well-coordinated way.

Step by Step Instructions

1. Sit on the chair, place your feet flat on the floor, arms at your sides
2. Extend your right leg forward and place your right heel on the floor. At the same time extend your right arm in front of you, elbow straight
3. Hold this position for about 3 seconds
4. Return to the starting position and repeat the same movement with your left arm and leg

Tips and Tricks

I suggest you do this exercise slowly a couple of times before starting it to be able to perfectly understand the movement you need to conduct. When you are getting into it, you could repeat it in a controlled way without issues.

Breathing

Keep your breathing slow and controlled.

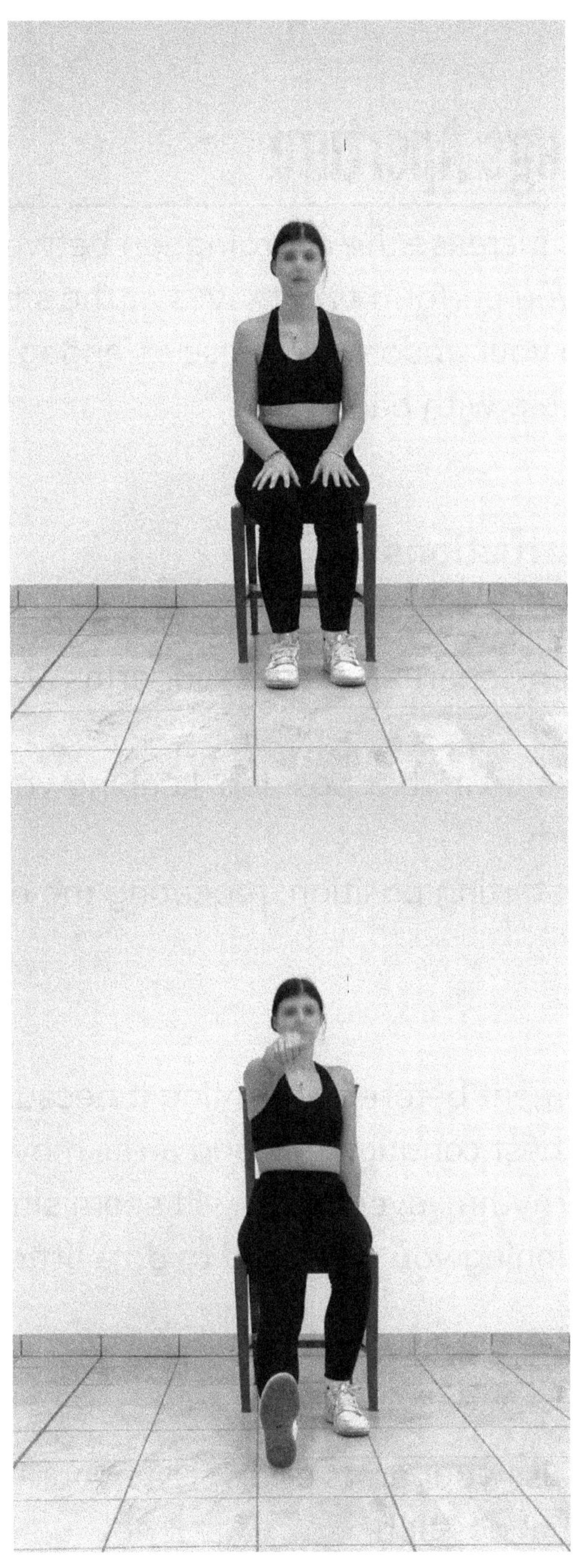

22 Lifting + Legs Aperture

This exercise helps increase the coordination between mind and muscle by having you perform two moves at the same time. Remember to keep your abdominal muscles engaged during the entire exercise to help with balance.

Step by Step Instructions

1. Sit on the chair, placing your feet on the floor
2. Spread your legs apart and raise your arms above your head at the same time
3. Hold your arms up in that position, keeping your legs apart, for about 3 seconds
4. Return to the starting position, repeating the exercise

Tips and Tricks

Focus on the movement before performing it because coordination will be required to best conduct legs and arms movement. When you find your personal rhythm, everything will seem simple and more natural. At the beginning you will need to do a little practice.

Breathing

Exhale when you raise your arms and spread your legs, inhale upon returning to the initial position.

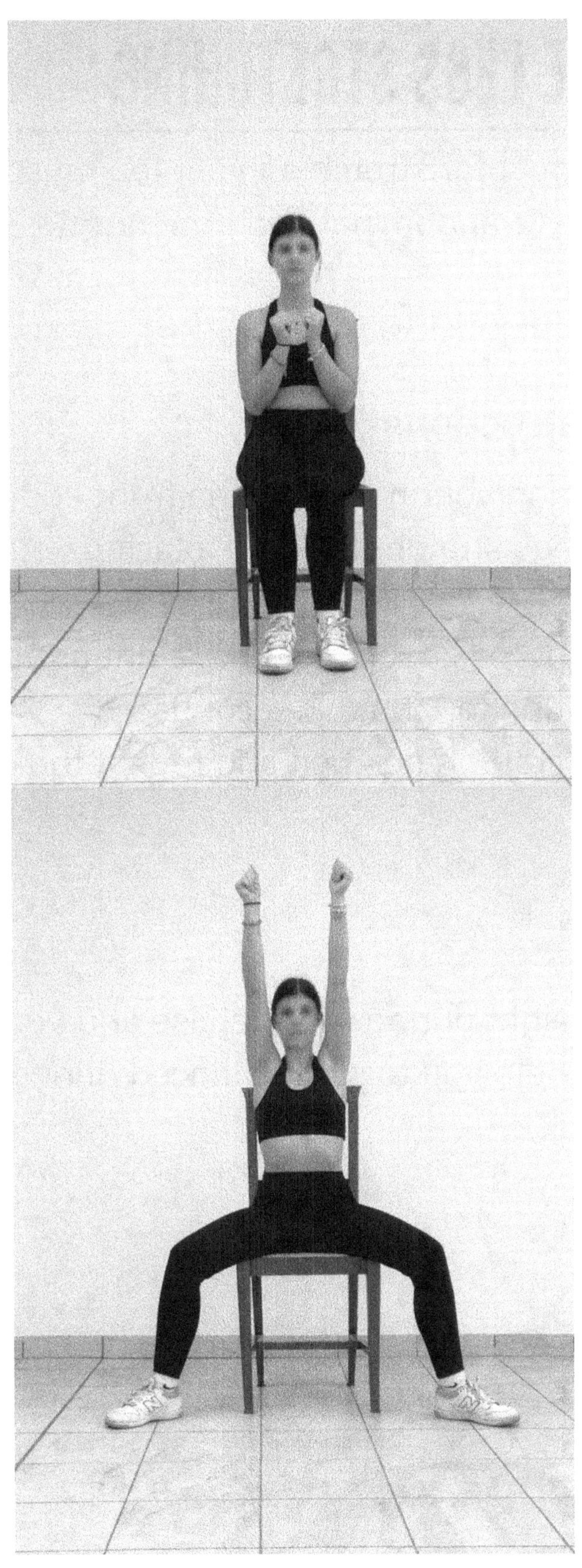

23 ALTERNATE LEGS STRETCHING

This exercise is perfect for stretching your leg muscles, especially your hamstrings. Your abdominal and arm muscles will also be involved.

Step by Step Instructions

1. Sit down, placing your hands on the front edge of the chair
2. Extend your legs straight forward, placing your heels on the floor
3. Raise your right leg keeping it as straight as you can
4. Hold this position for about 3 seconds
5. Return to the starting position and repeat the exercise with the other leg

Tips and Tricks

Keep your back straight during the exercise and your hands firmly on the chair. This will help you to stay balanced during the entire exercise.

Breathing

Keep your breathing slow and controlled.

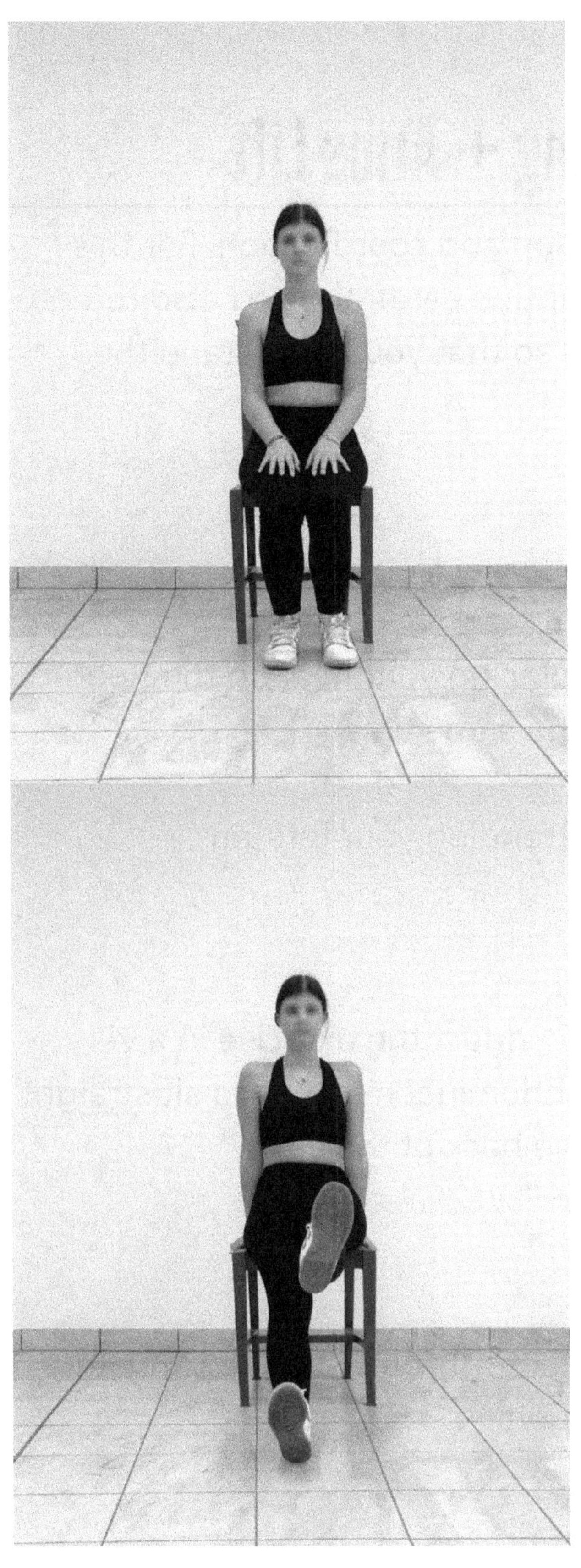
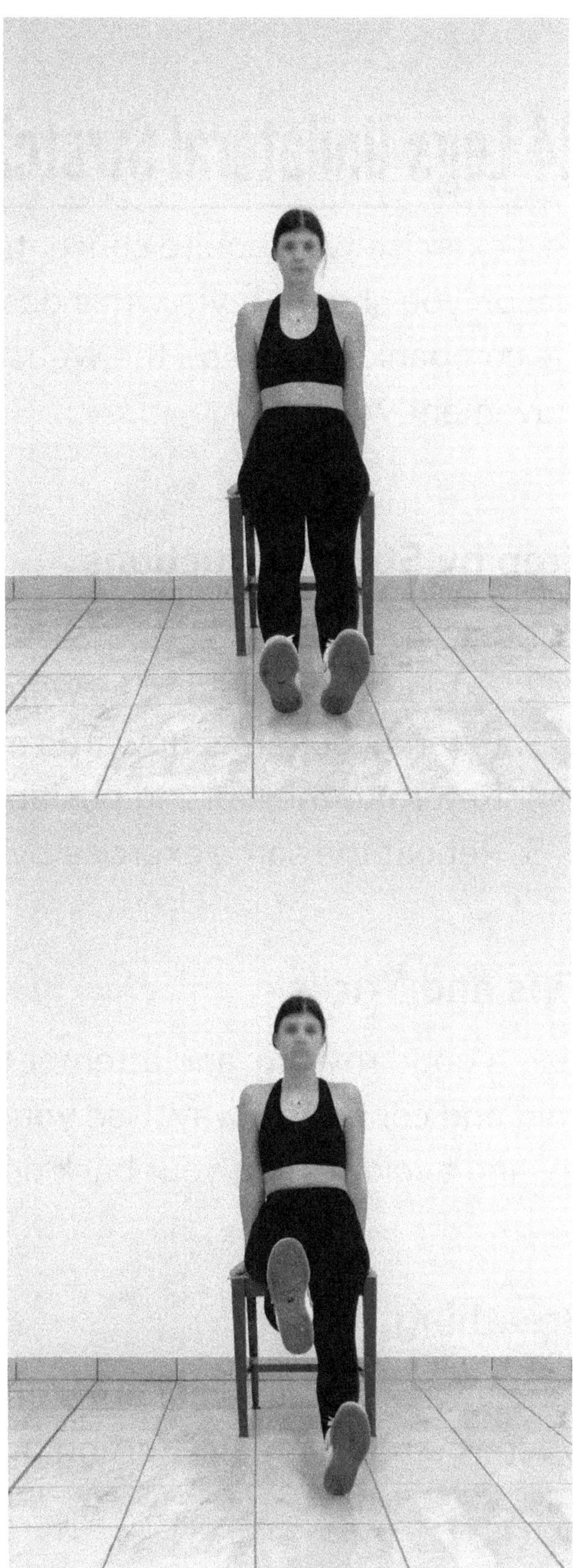

24 Legs Unilateral Stretching + Arms Lift

This exercise will require concentration and coordination. For this reason you should review this description carefully, and also refer to the companion video on the website so that you understand the movement well.

Step by Step Instructions

1. Sit on the chair
2. Extend your right leg forward, placing your heel on the floor
3. Extend your arms upwards at the same time
4. Return to the starting position
5. Repeat the same exercise by extending your left leg

Tips and Tricks

Find a good rhythm, and attempt to conduct the exercise in a very fluid and controlled way. Use your abdominal muscles to sit straight up, and avoid resting your back on the back of the chair.

Breathing

Exhale when you lift your arms and extend your leg. Then, inhale when you return to the starting position.

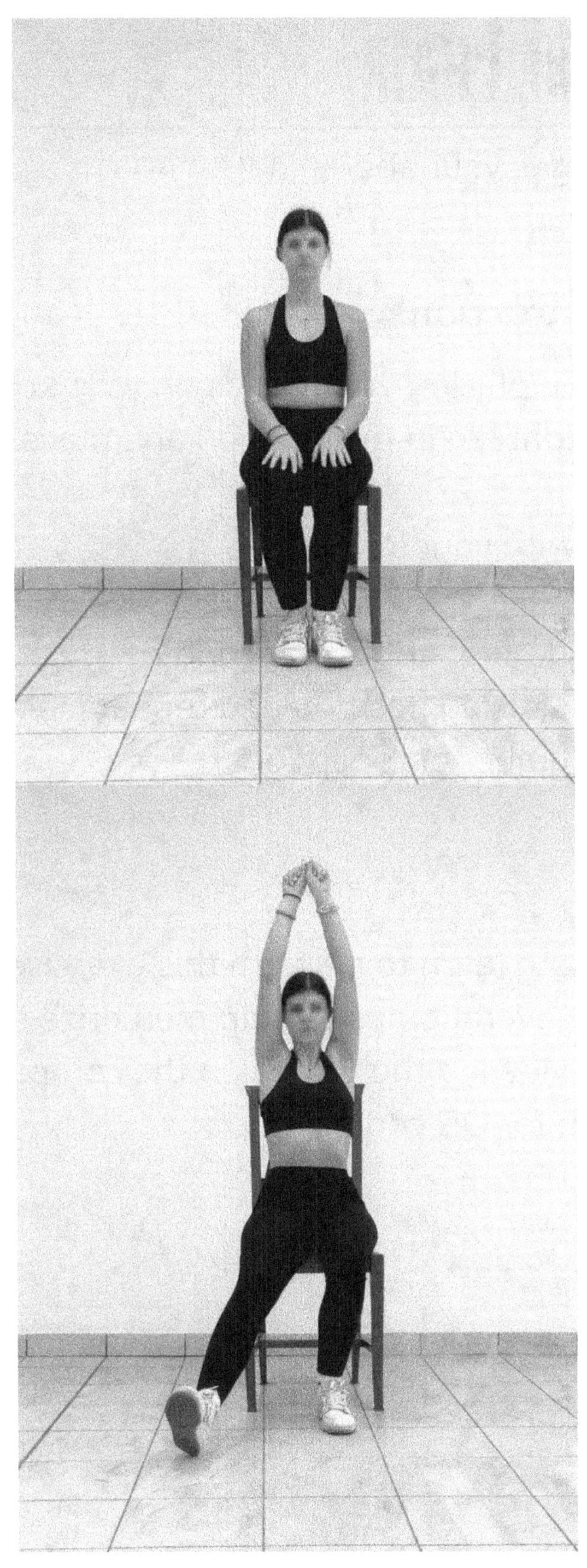

25 FROG ON THE CHAIR

This exercise engages your abdominals.

Step by Step Instructions

1. Sit on the chair, placing your hands on your knees
2. Extend your right leg in front of you and place your right heel on the floor
3. Do the same with your left leg
4. Now, lift both your knees up to your chest at the same time
5. Hold this position for about 3 seconds
6. Return to the starting position and repeat (see the day by day program for number of repetitions)

Tips and Tricks

It may take practice to learn to perform this exercise smoothly. Reading this page several times to help memorize the movements will help, as will reviewing the videos on the companion website (see introduction section for QR code).

Breathing

Exhale when you bring your knees to your chest and inhale when you straighten your legs.

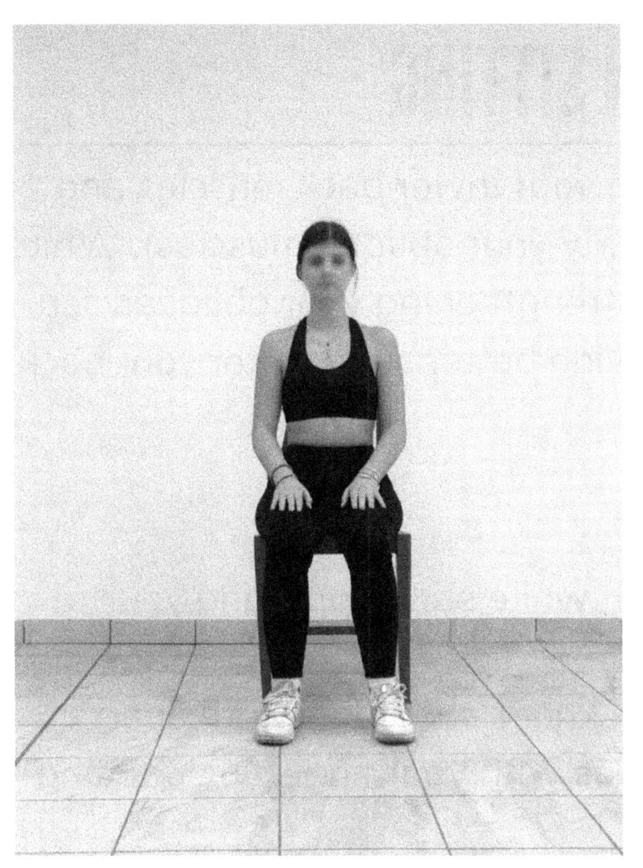 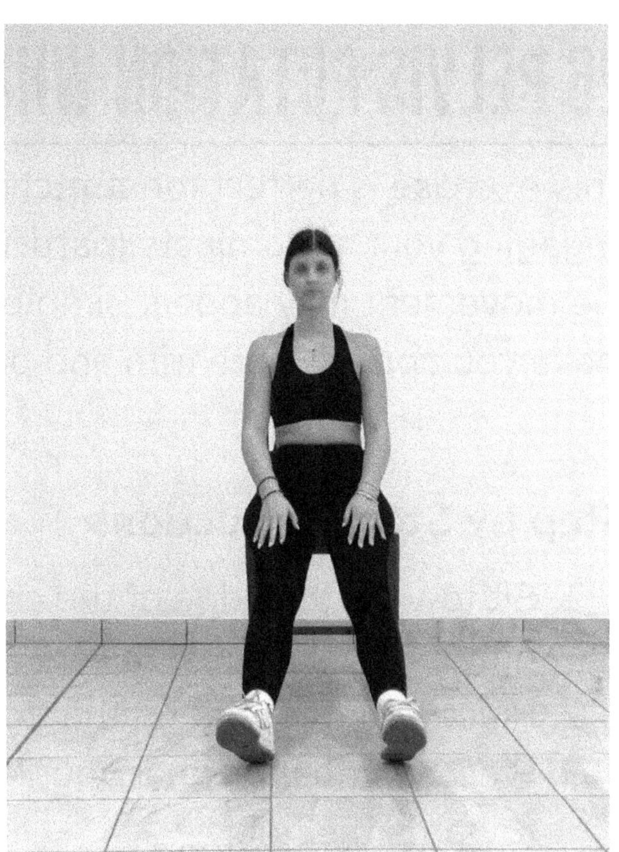

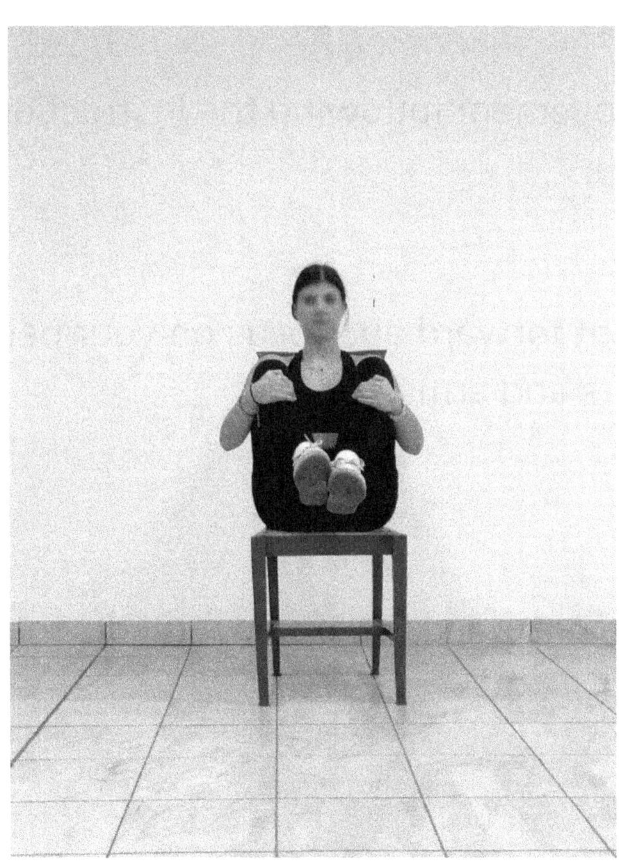

26 PELVIS ROTATION WHEN SITTING

This exercise is perfect for stretching your lower back muscles and engaging your abdominals (particularly your oblique muscles). While the movement may appear simple, strengthening your obliques can make you appear more trim and provide better support for your back.

Step by Step Instructions

1. Sit toward the edge of the chair, while still supporting your glutes
2. Place your feet flat on the floor, knees shoulder width apart
3. Place your hands near your knees with your fingertips pointing towards the floor
4. Smoothly rotate your pelvis 360 ° pelvis rotation without pausing
5. Repeat the movement following the instructions in the program

Tips and Tricks

Stare at a fixed point forward and focus on your pelvis movement, relax your shoulders and arms.

Breathing

Maintain slow and controlled breathing, and do not hold your breath.

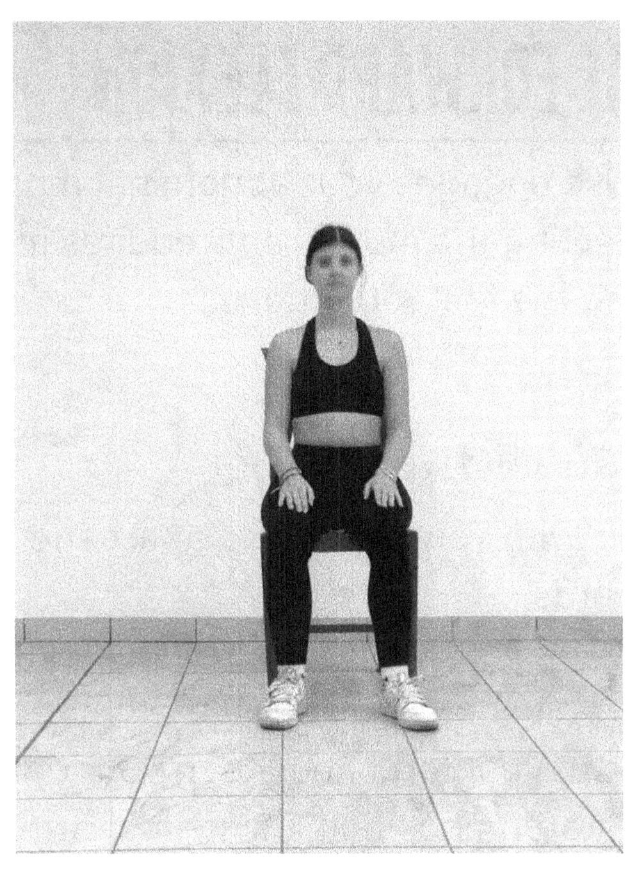

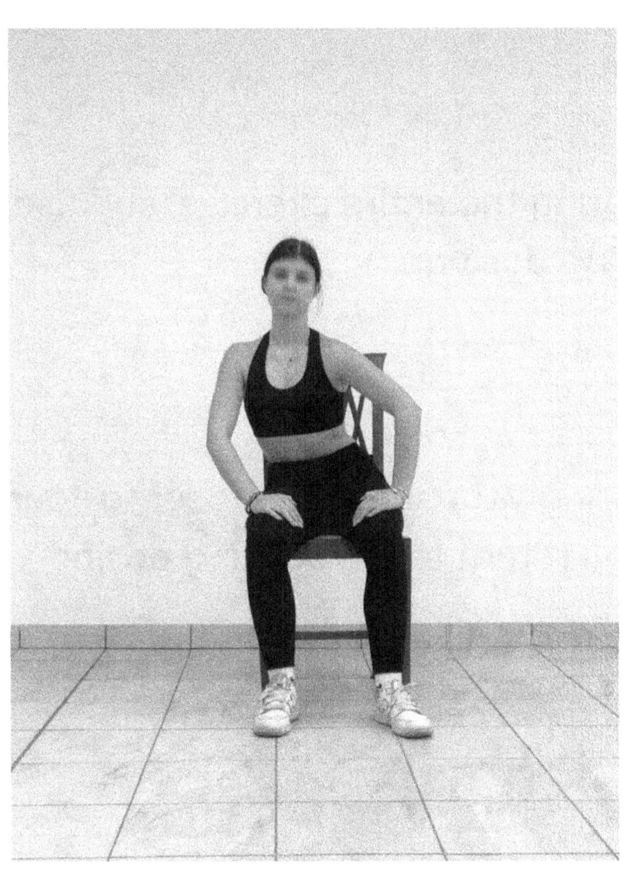

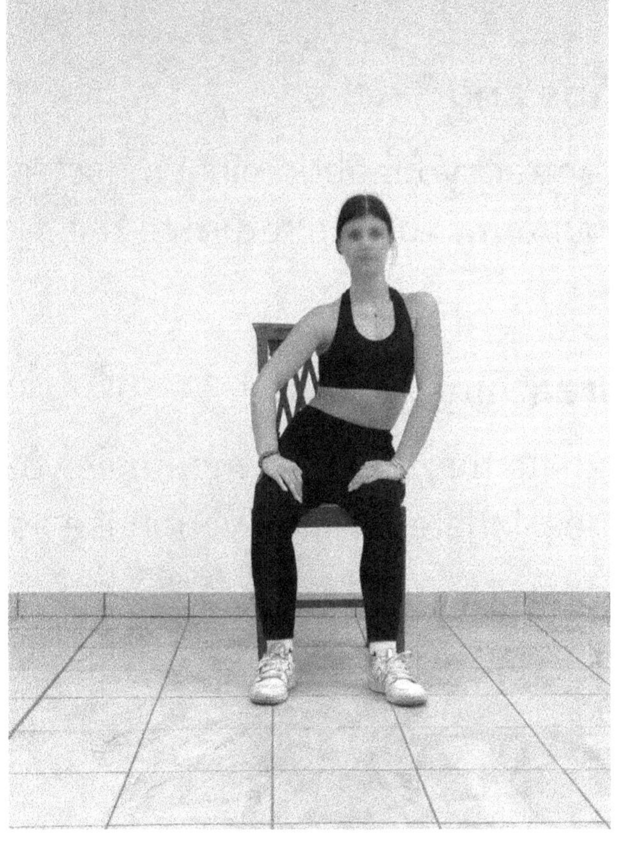

27 UNILATERAL FORWARD FLEXION

This mobility exercise engages your abdominal musles, especially your obliques. Perfecting the movement requires attention and concentration during the first repetitions.

Step by Step Instructions

1. Sit on the chair with your legs wide apart and your toes by pointing outwards
2. Put your hands on your thighs, fingertips pointing down
3. Lean forward while bending your left elbow to bring your right shoulder close to your left knee. Keep your right arm straight
4. Return to the starting position, using your arms to help
5. Conduct the same movement on the opposite side

Tips and Tricks

Contract your abdominal muscles during the entire exercise, and use your arms to help return to the starting position.

Breathing

Exhale through your mouth as you bring your shoulder closer to your knee. Inhale through your nose as you return to the starting position.

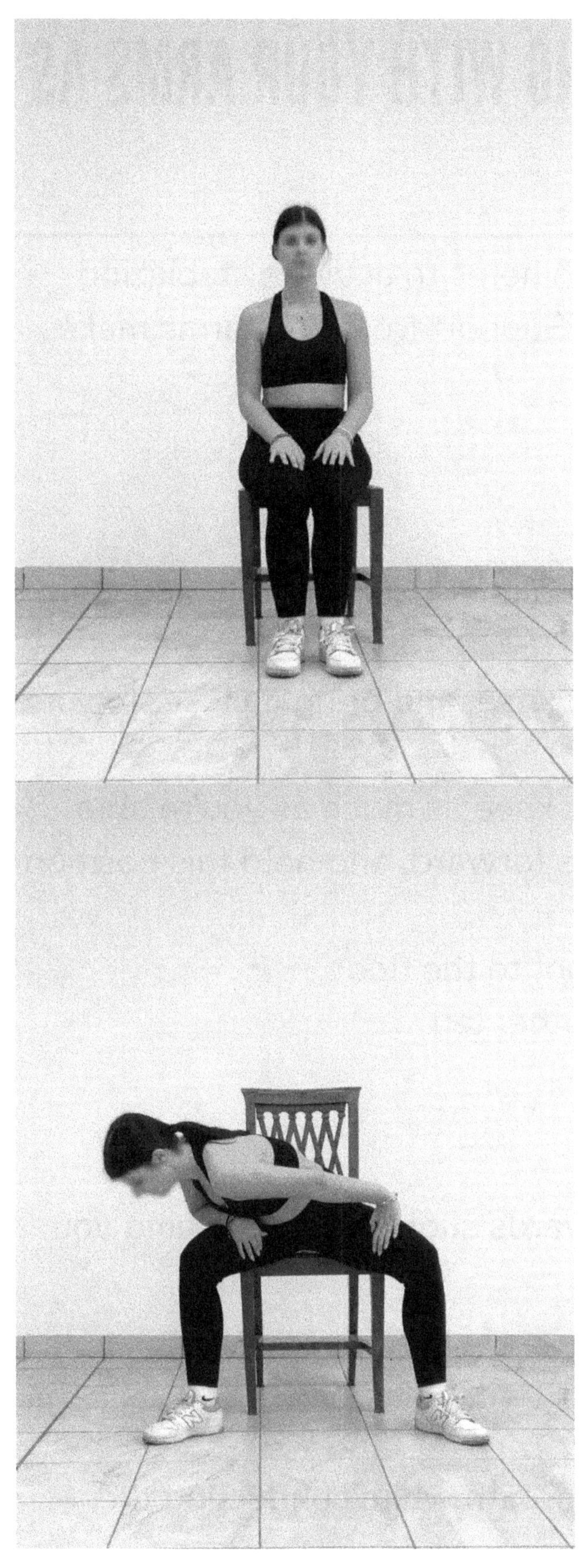
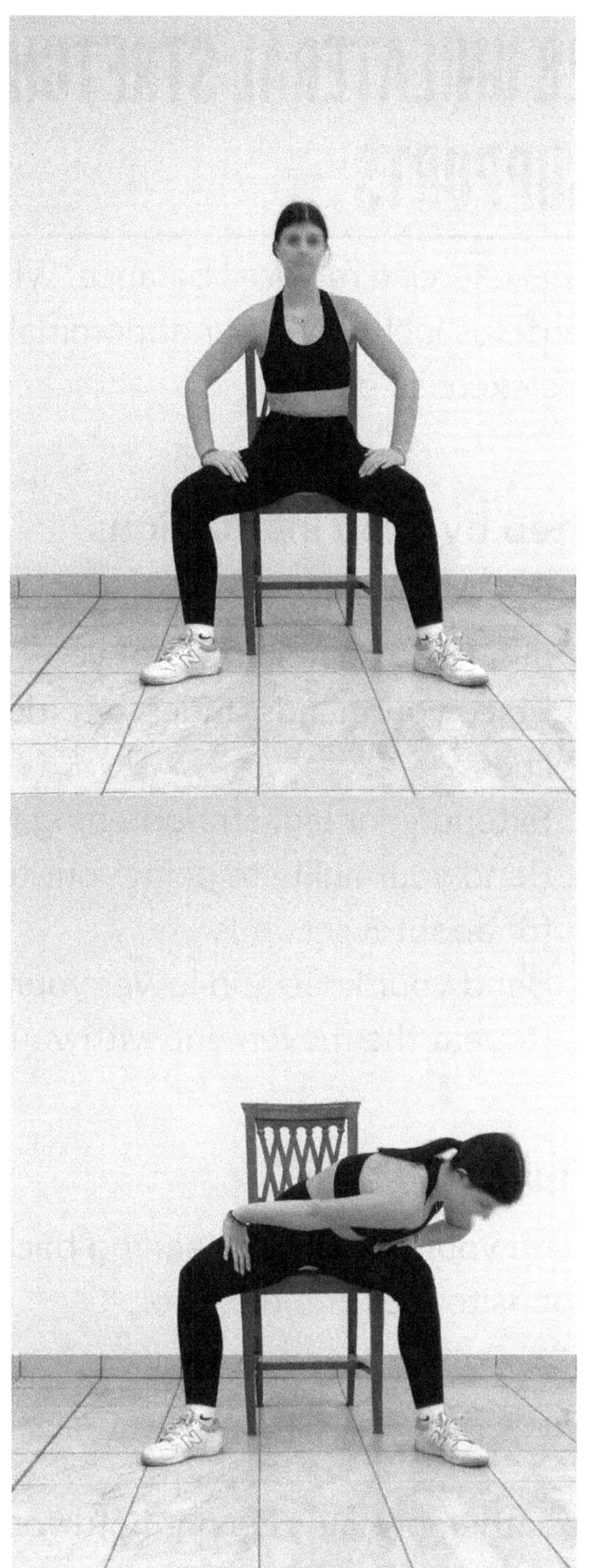

28 UNILATERAL STRETCHING WITH YOUR ARMS AS SUPPORTS

This exercise requires balance, which helps to activate stabilizing muscles including your abdominals. Support from your arms makes the exercise easier.

Step by Step Instructions

1. Sit on the edge of the chair, keeping your back straight, and stare at a fixed point in front of you
2. Place your hands under your right knee, and bring it closer to your chest
3. Extend your leg, straightening the knee as much as you're able
4. Bend your ankle to point your toes forward, and hold this position for about 3 seconds
5. Bend your knee and lower your foot to the floor
6. Repeat the movement with your other leg

Tips and Tricks

Keep your balance by leaning backwards slightly, and pushing your opposite foot into the floor.

Breathing

Breathe normally. Do not hold your breath while conducting the exercise.

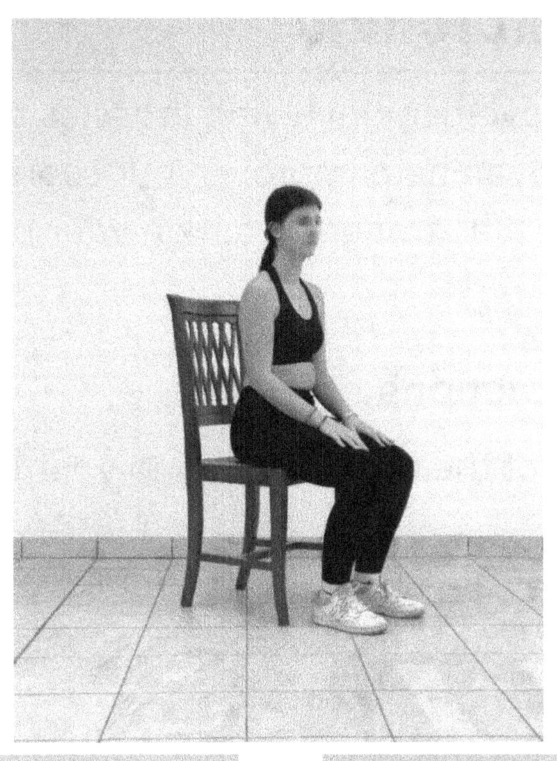

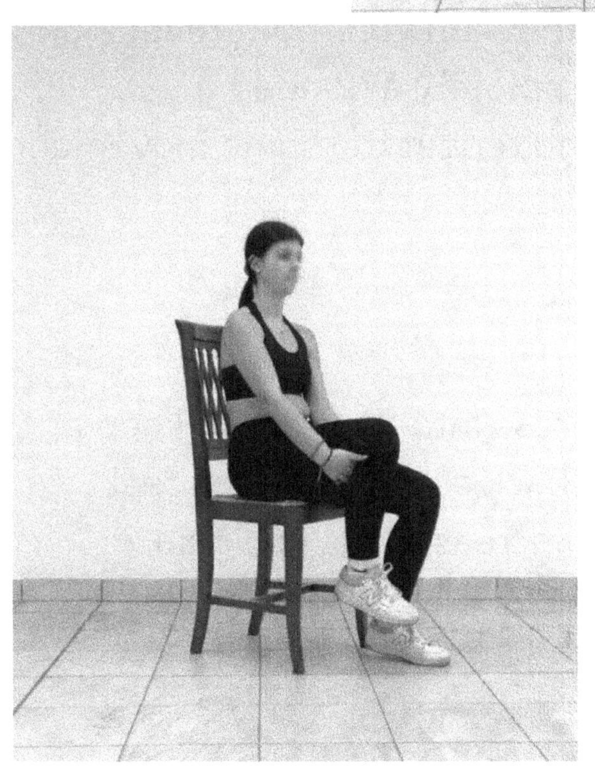

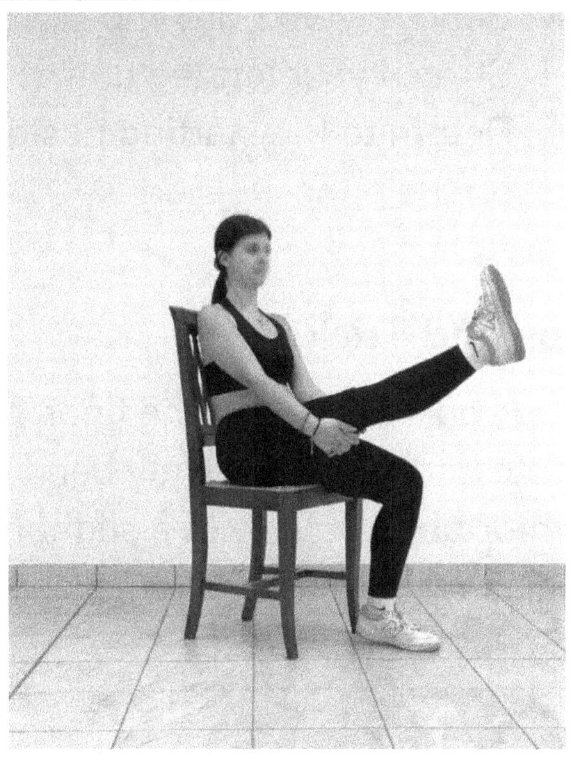

29 LATERAL STRETCHING

This is a complete movement involving muscles that are not frequently worked. It can help improve your coordination and spinal flexibility. You will feel a strong stretch on your back.

Step by Step Instructions

1. Sit on the edge of the chair, spreading your legs and toes outwards
2. Extend your arms at your sides and relax
3. Place your right hand on your abdomen, raising your left arm above your head
4. Bend to your right and put the elbow on your right thigh
5. Stretch your left leg until it is completely extended
6. Return to the starting position and repeat the same movement on the opposite side

Tips and Tricks

Keep your feet flat on the floor, and press into the floor to keep a stable body position. Only bend your back as much as you feel comfortable. Start with a slight bend, increasing as you gain familiarity with the movement.

Breathing

Exhale through your mouth when you bend sideways and inhale through your nose when you return to the starting position.

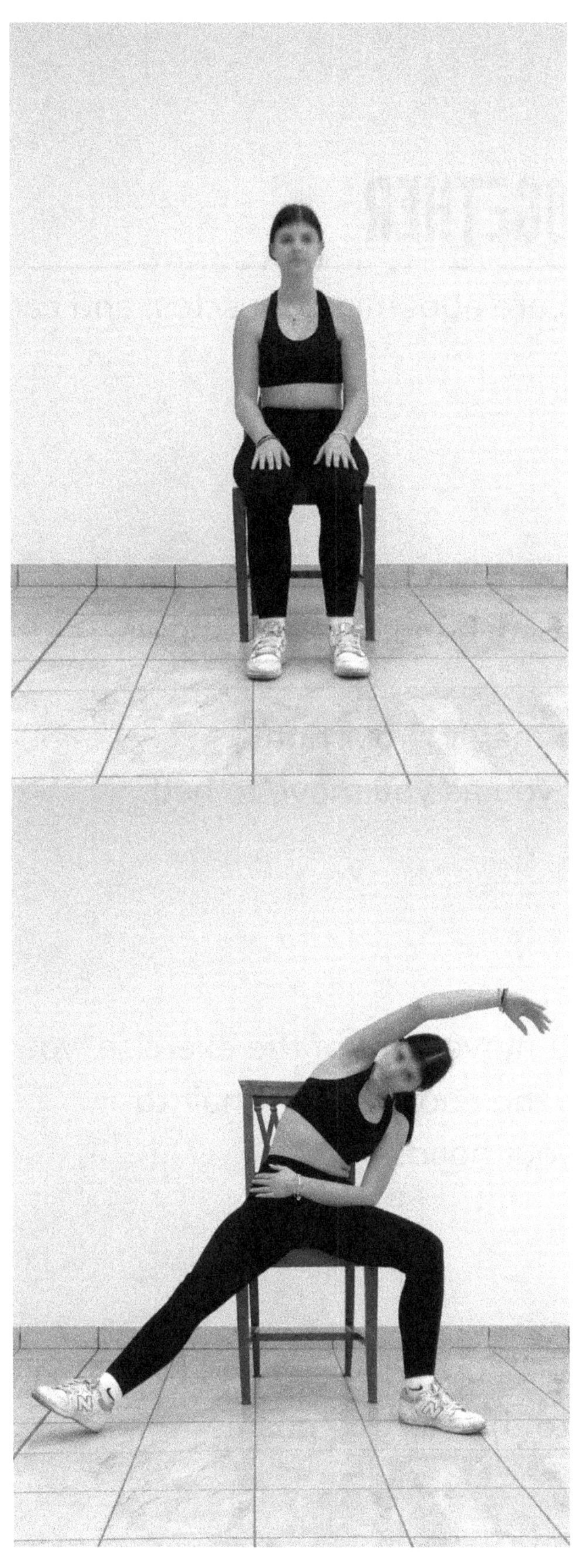

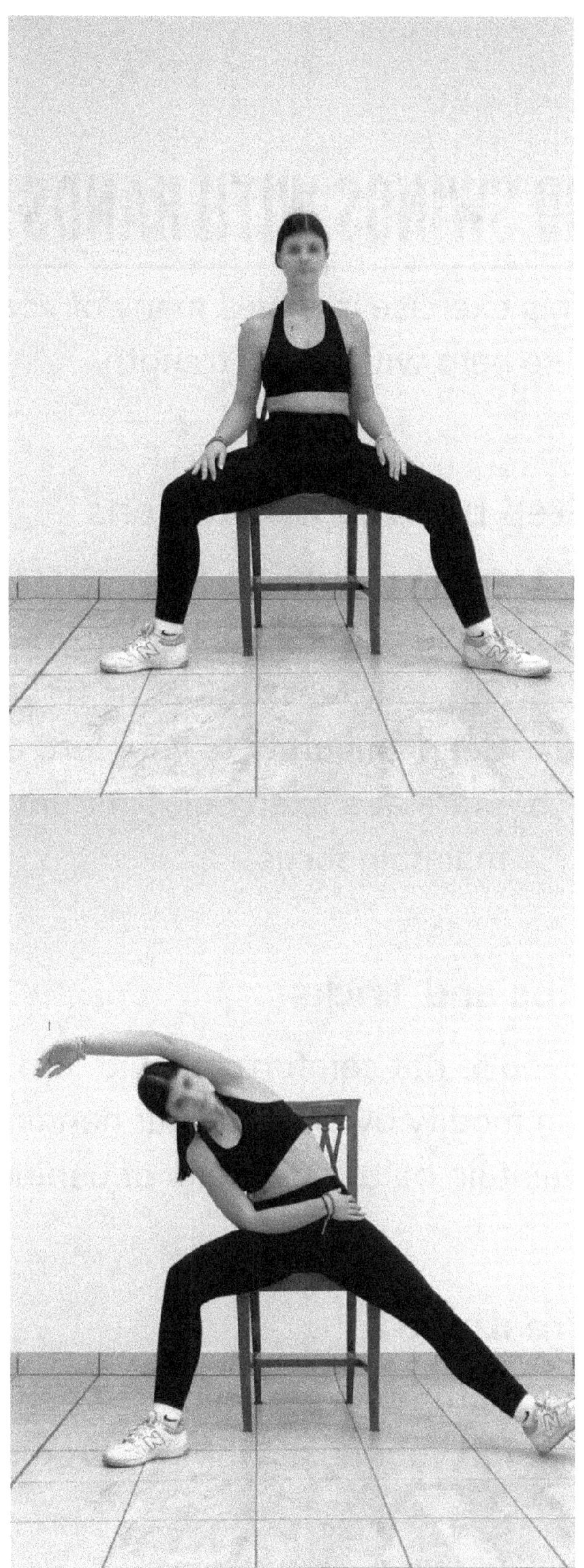

30 SWINGS WITH HANDS TOGETHER

This exercise involves many of your core abdominal muscles, and can also help with back strength.

Step by Step Instructions

1. Sit on the chair, placing your arms at your sides
2. Bring your hands behind your head, bending your elbows
3. Put your feet flat on the floor
4. Bend smoothly to your left, and then to your right
5. Stare at a fixed point in front of you as you move to help maintain focus

Tips and Tricks

If you're not comfortable with the full movement of the exercise, you can modify by placing your hands on the edges of the chair to maintain balance instead of behind your head.

Breathing

Exhale through your mouth when you bend sideways and then inhale through your nose when you return to the starting position.

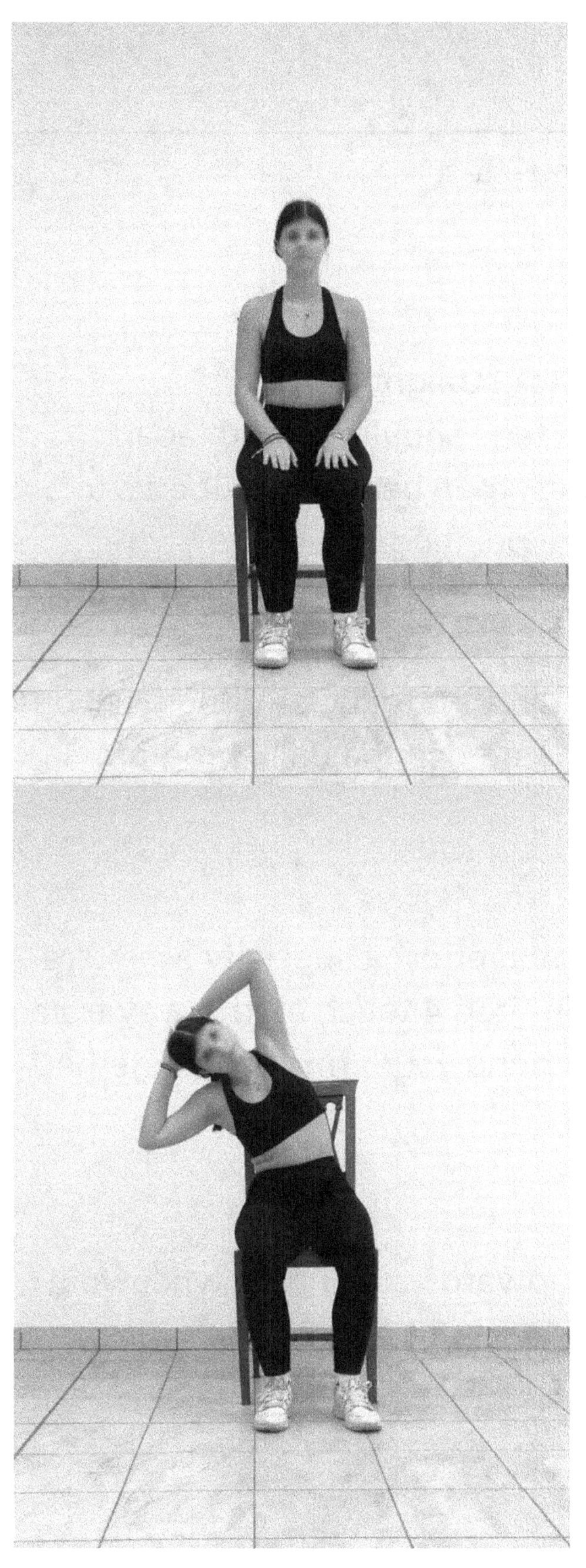

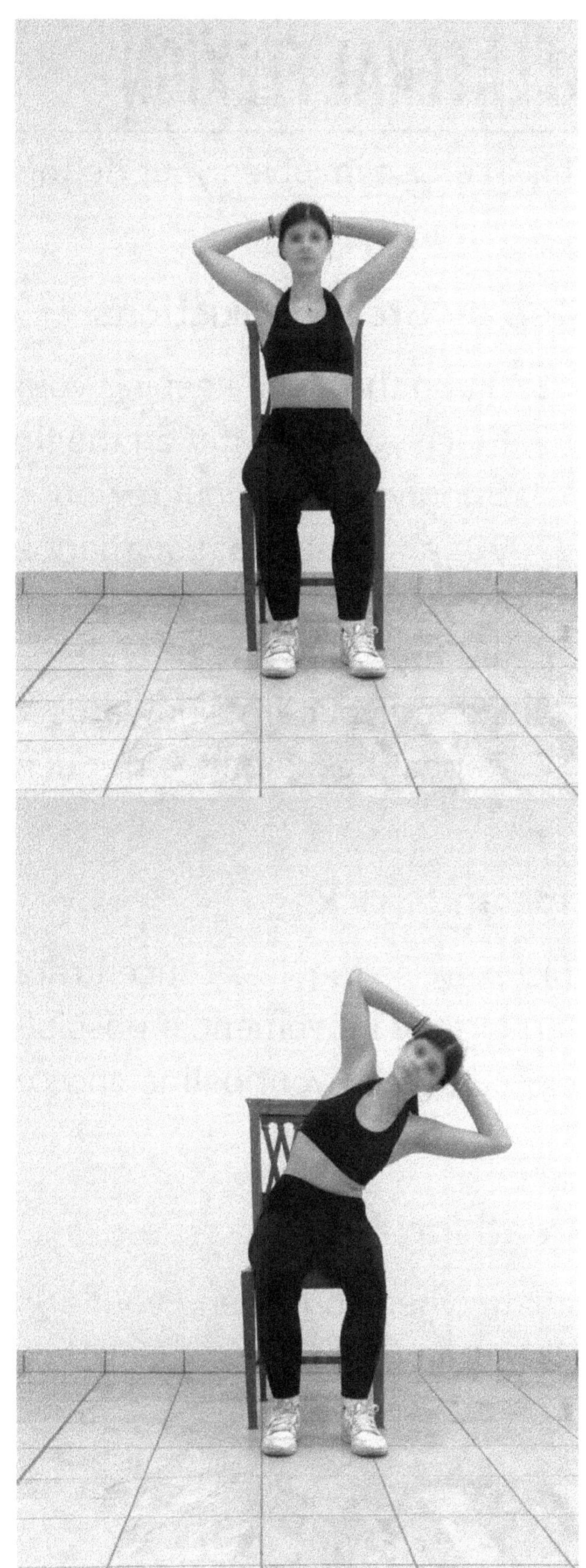

31 LATERAL FLEXION

This exercise involves your deltoid muscles.

Step by Step Instructions

1. Sit on the chair, keeping your back straight
2. Place your feet flat on the floor, legs shoulder width apart
3. Bring your arms out to your sides, then bend your elbows to a 90° angle so that your hands are pointing up
4. Move your bent arms together in front of you until your palms are touching
5. Extend your arms upwards, then return to the starting position
6. Repeat based on the frequency stated in the daily program

Tips and Tricks

This exercise requires concentration and effort, especially as you're learning the movement. If possible, in Step 4 touch all the way from your elbows to your palms once you bring your arms back together.

Breathing

Exhale when you extend your arms upwards and inhale when you return to the starting position.

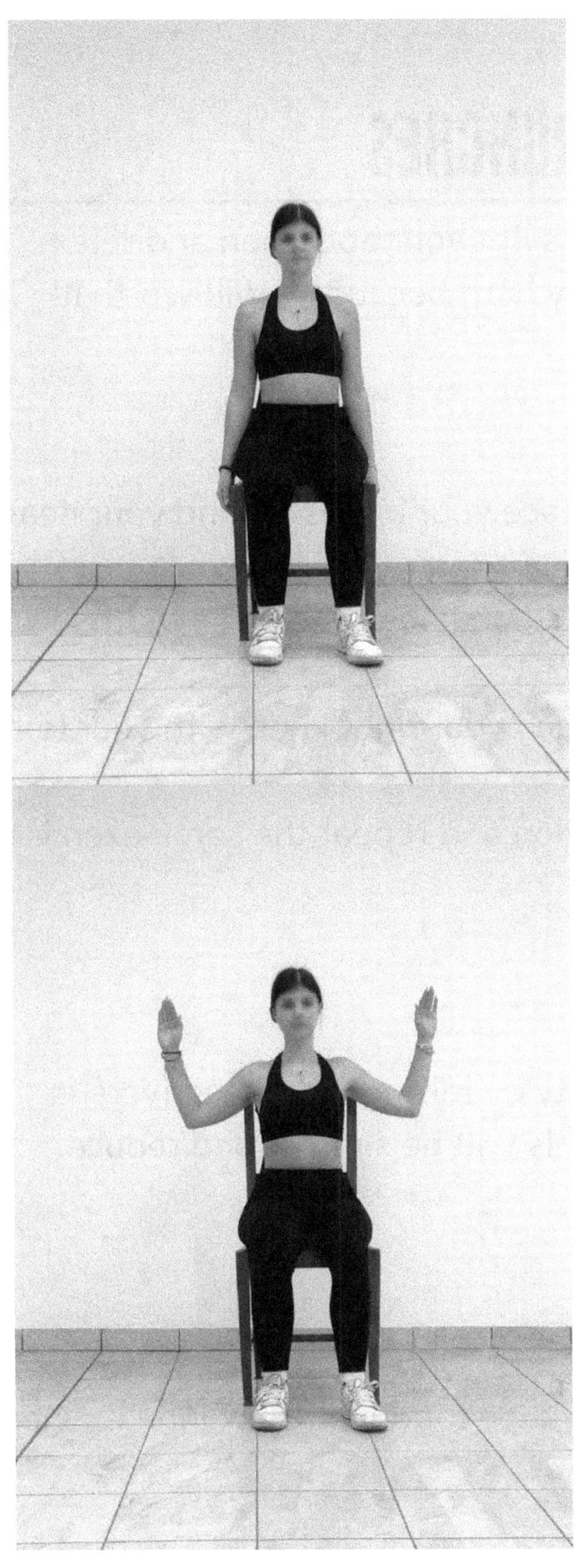
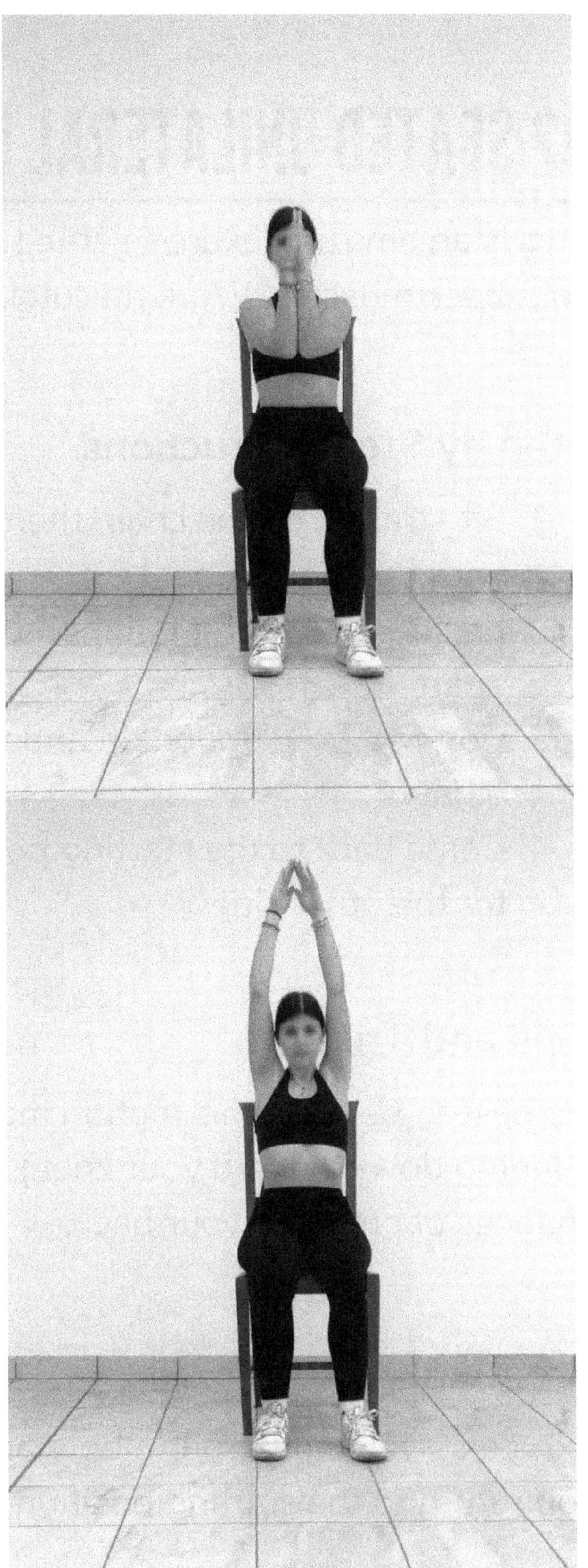

32 SEATED UNILATERAL CRUNCHES

This is an amazing exercise able to sculpt your abdomen and relax your back muscles. Work ridiculously hard because it will worth it!

Step by Step Instructions

1. Sit straight on the chair, then place your hands behind your head with the elbows bent
2. Ensure your feet are flat on the floor, knees shoulder width apart
3. Contract your abdomen and touch your right knee with your left elbow
4. Come back to the starting position and repeat the same exercise for the other side

Tips and Tricks

It's best to perform this motion mainly by raising your knee (versus bending down toward your knee). This will be simpler and reduce chances of straining your back.

Breathing

Exhale as you move your elbow and knee together, then, inhale when you return to the starting position.

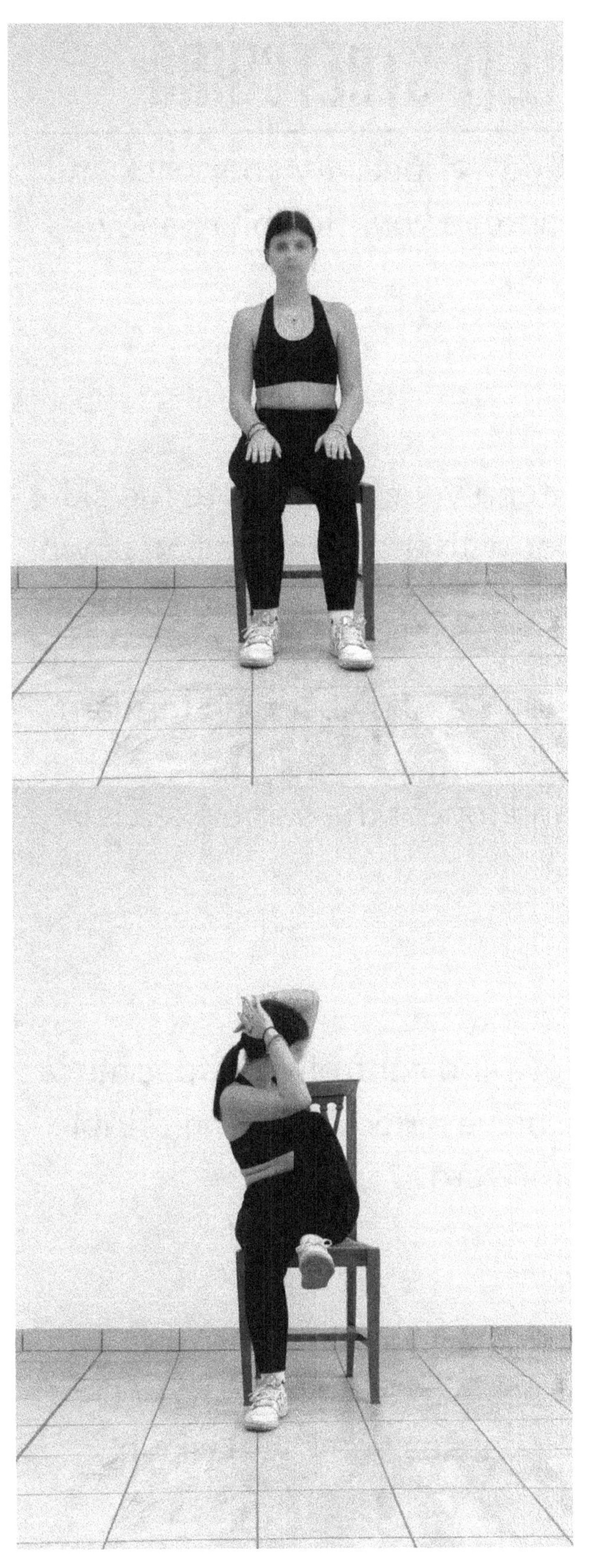
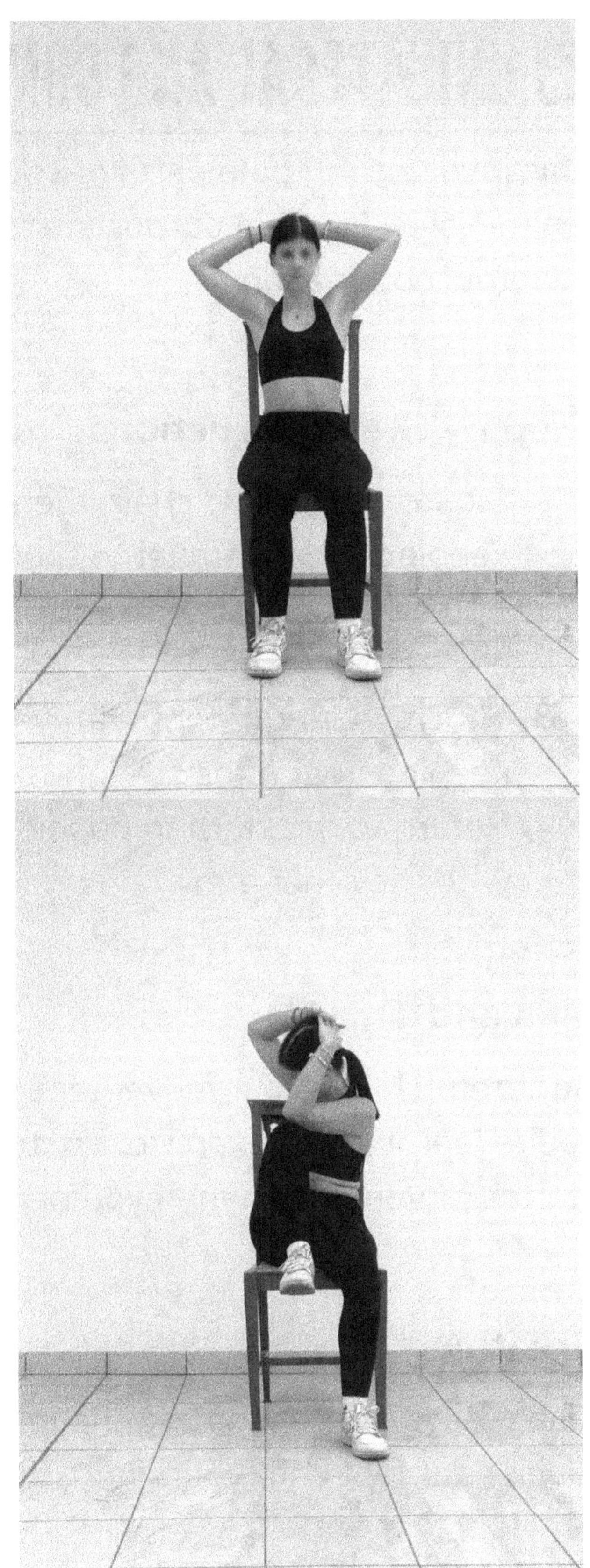

33 UNILATERAL AND COMPLETE STRETCHING

This involves multiple parts of your body, especially your back and leg muscles. Its main purpose is to improve your flexibility and general coordination.

Step by Step Instructions

1. Sit straight on the chair, then extend your arms out to the side, keeping them parallel to the floor with the palms facing down
2. Spread your legs and keep your feet as parallel to one another as possible
3. Touch your right foot with your left hand by bending forward, keeping your arms straight
4. Return to the starting position and repeat the same exercise with the other arm

Tips and Tricks

Be careful! Make your movements slow and controlled, especially as you're learning the exercise. Try to achieve a good but comfortable stretch of your back when you bend forward.

Breathing

Inhale when you are sitting the initial position, exhale when you touch your foot with your hand, then inhale as you rise back up.

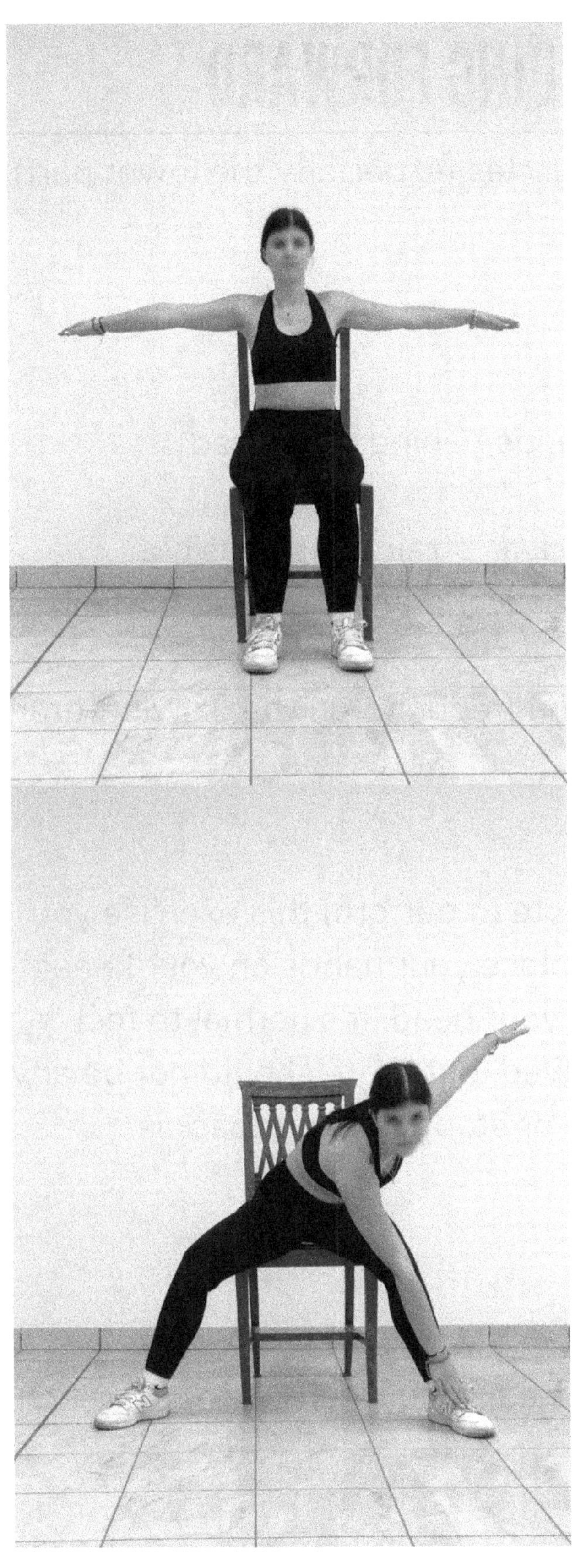
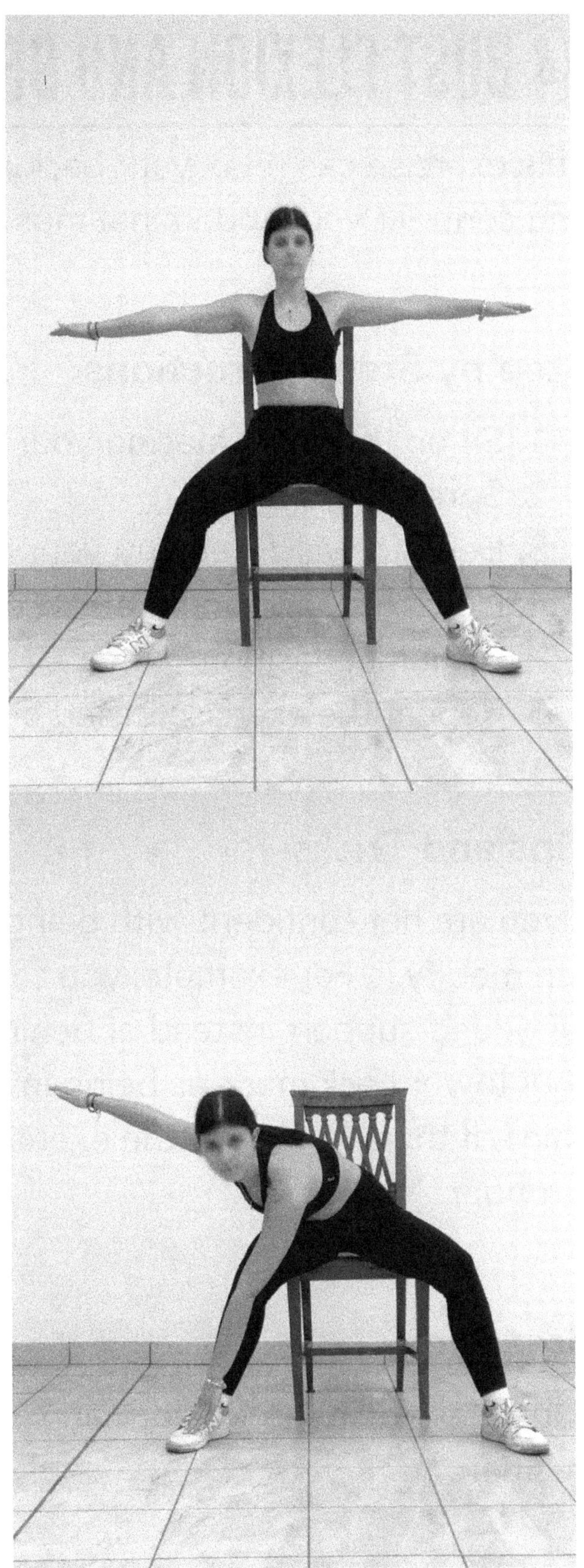

34 BUST FLEXION AND BENDING FORWARD

This exercise can relax your back muscles (especially the lower part) and contract your abdominal muscles.

Step by Step Instructions

1. Sit on the chair, placing your hands behind your head
2. Spread your legs
3. Bend forward, keeping your back as straight as possible
4. Hold this position for about one second and then rise back up to the initial position
5. Repeat the exercise based on the frequency in the daily program

Tips and Tricks

If you are not confident with being able to perform this exercise you can modify it. For example, you can place your hands on your knees for added support instead of behind your head. It's normal to feel your lower back muscles being involved, but there should not be any pain – if there is, modify the exercise or stop until your back is stronger.

Breathing

Exhale as you bend forward and inhale as you return to the starting position.

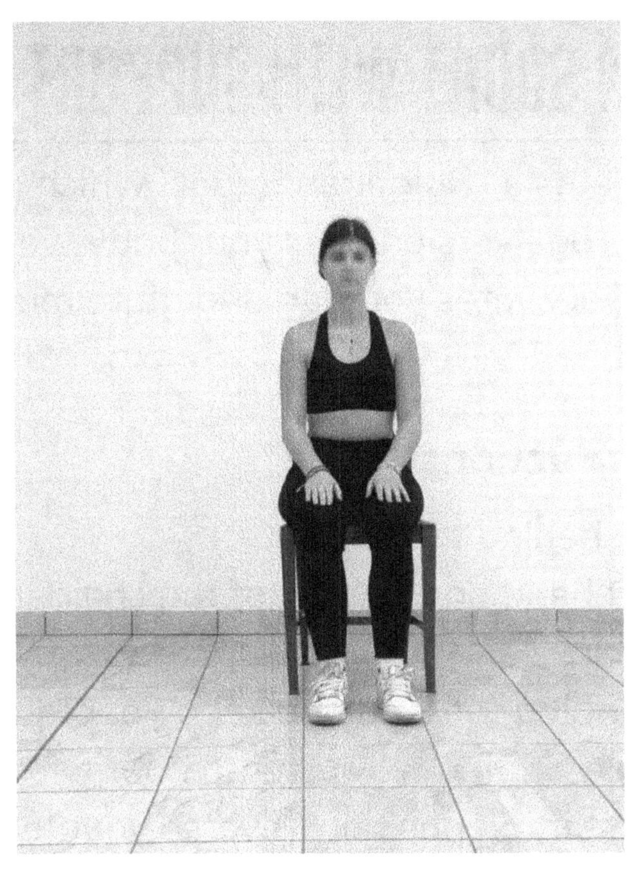

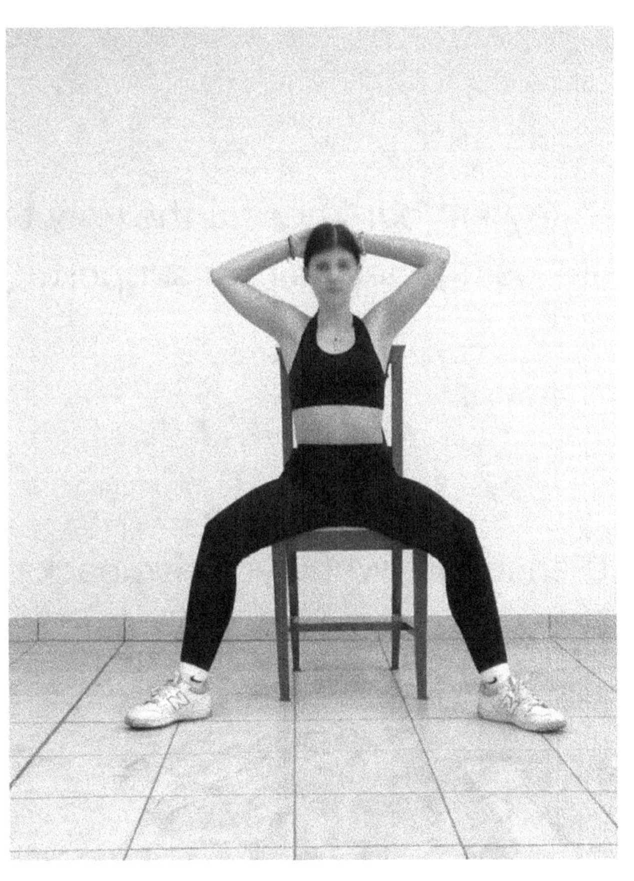

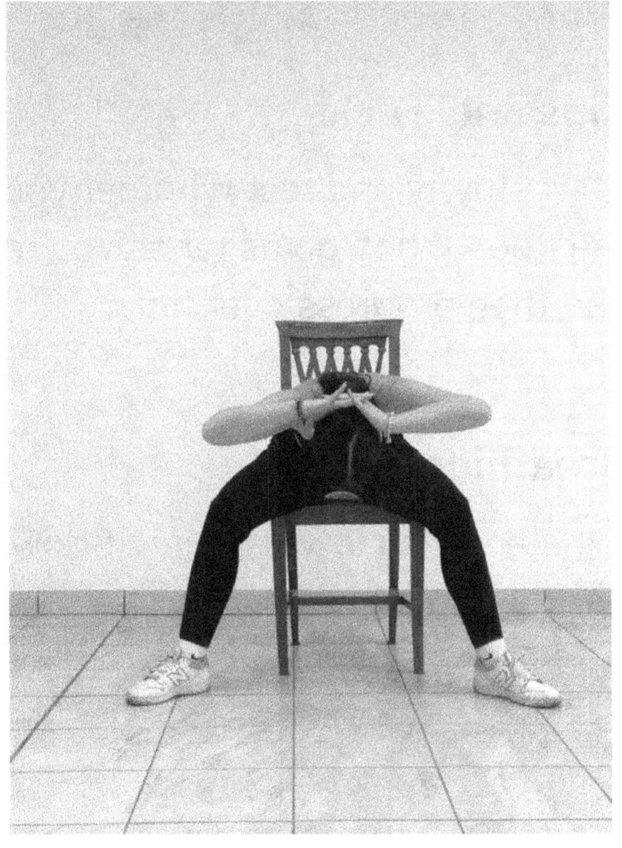

35 BULGARIAN SQUAT WITH SUPPORT

This exercise simulates a "Bulgarian Squat" which is often done with weight. This Chair Yoga version uses your body weight only, with the chair assisting, and activates your leg and glute muscles.

Step by Step Instructions

1. Stand directly behind the chair
2. Place your left hand on the back of the chair and your right hand on your right hip
3. Bring your right leg forward and keep your left leg back
4. Bend your knees, trying to touch the floor with your left knee
5. Return to the starting position, reverse your legs and hands, and repeat the exercise

Tips and Tricks

Start slowly and test whether you can lower your knee all the way to the floor. If not, go as far as you're able, using the chair for support, and then progress over time.

Breathing

Exhale as you lower yourself down, then inhale when you rise back up.

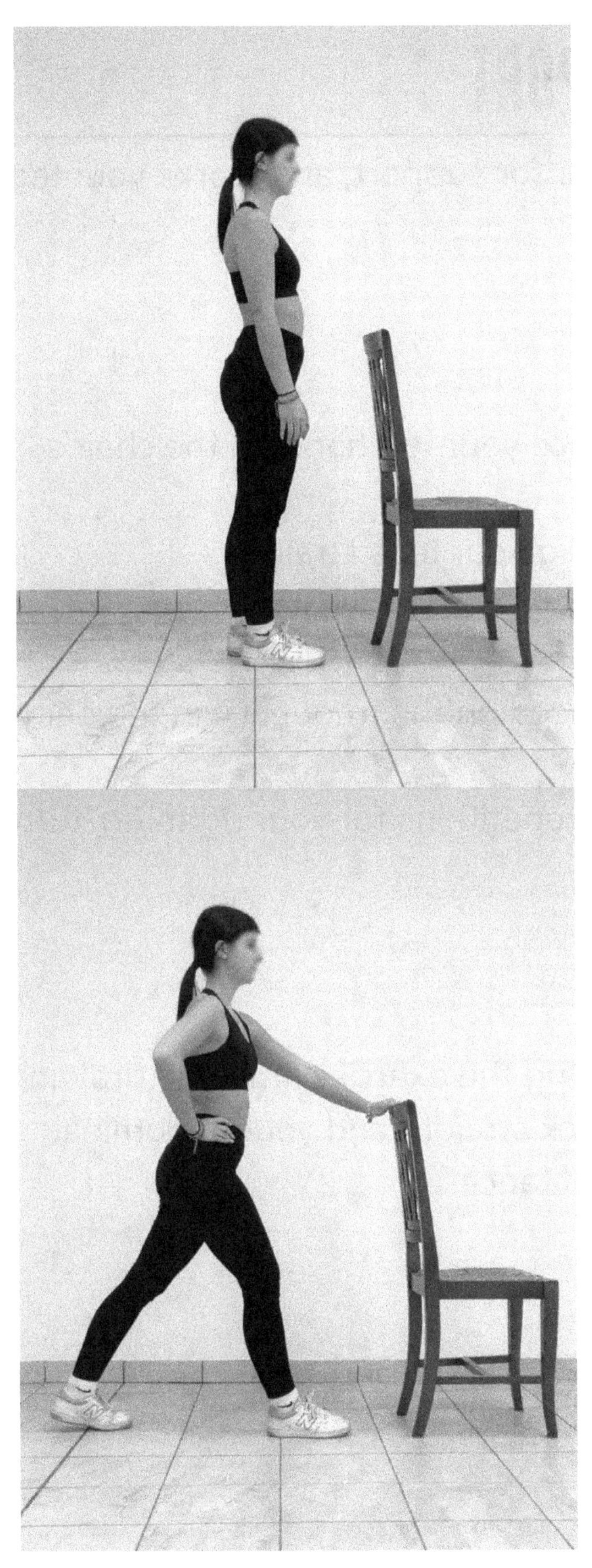
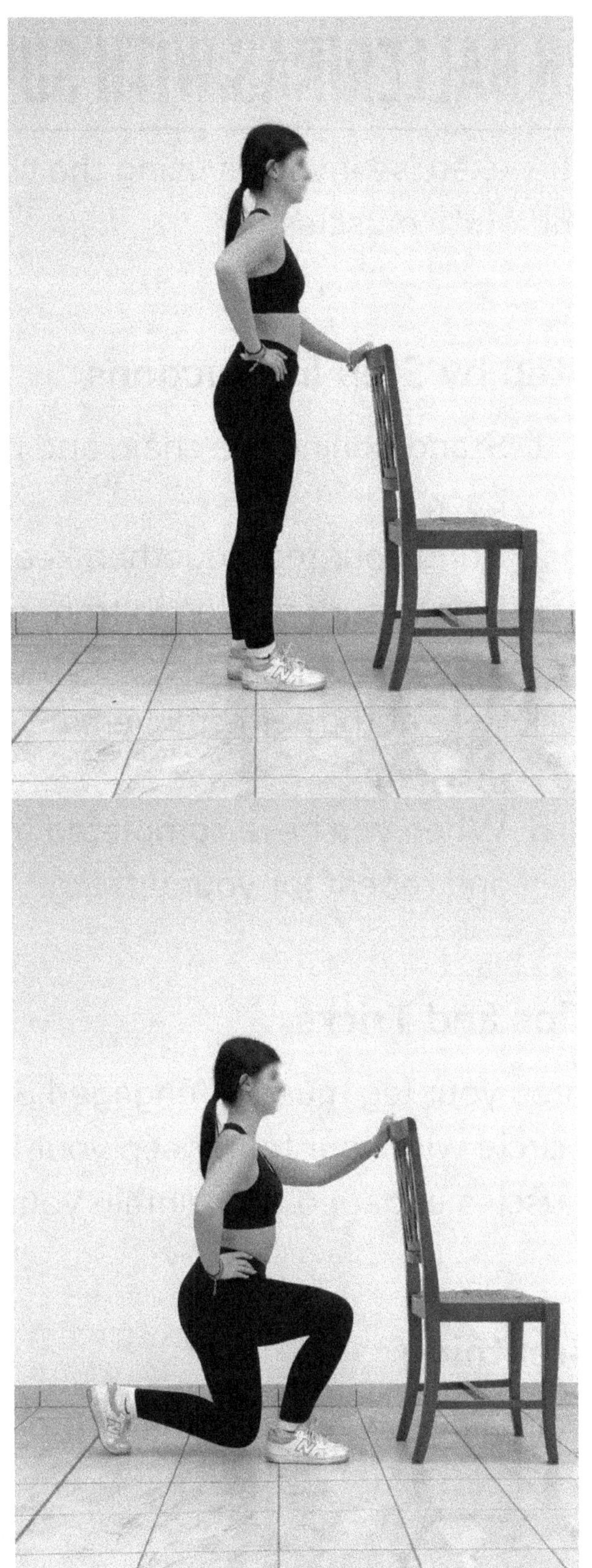

36 BALLERINAS WITH SUPPORT

This exercise involves using the chair for support, and works your leg and glute muscles.

Step by Step Instructions

1. Stand behind the chair, and place your left hand on the chair's back
2. Bring your feet together, keeping your legs straight
3. Raise your right leg in front of you, then move it in a circular motion
4. Repeat the same movement based on the frequency in the daily program
5. When you have completed all repetitions for your right leg, turn and repeat for your left leg

Tips and Tricks

Keep your leg muscles engaged during the exercise. Imagine drawing a circle with your foot. Keep your back straight and your abdominal muscles engaged to maintain your balance.

Breathing

Maintain slow and controlled breathing.

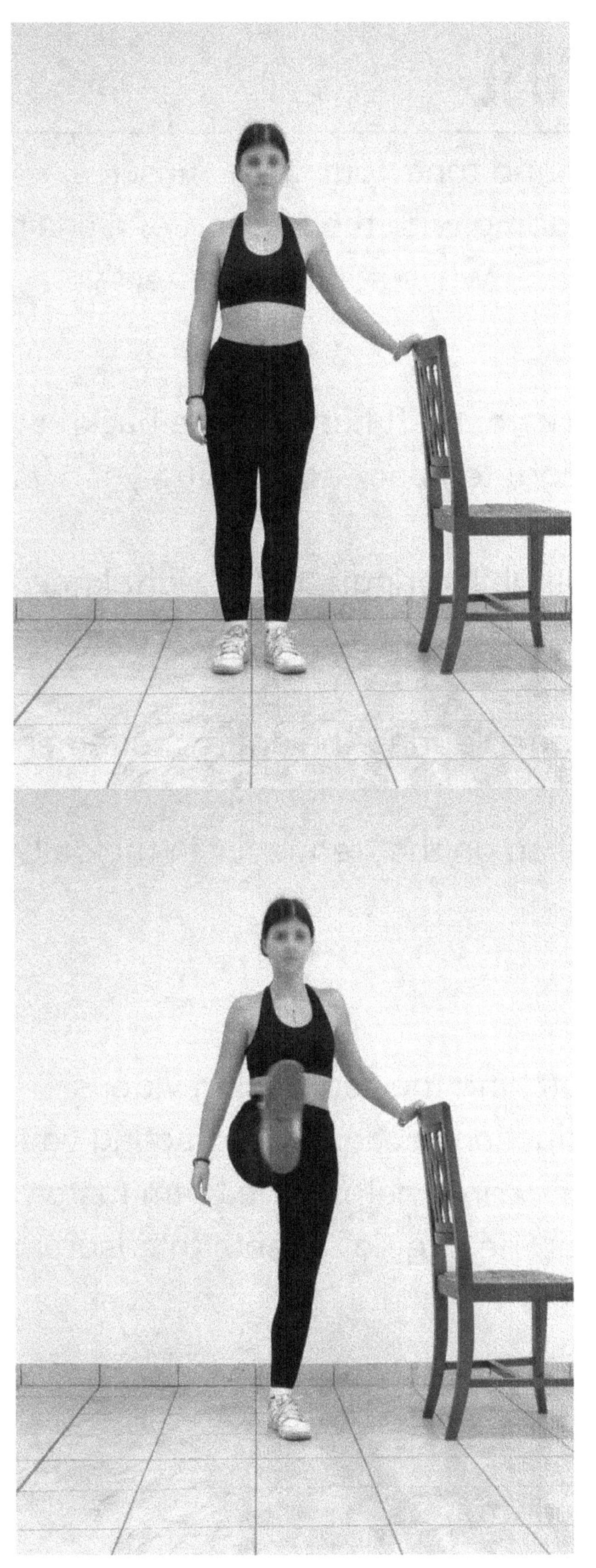

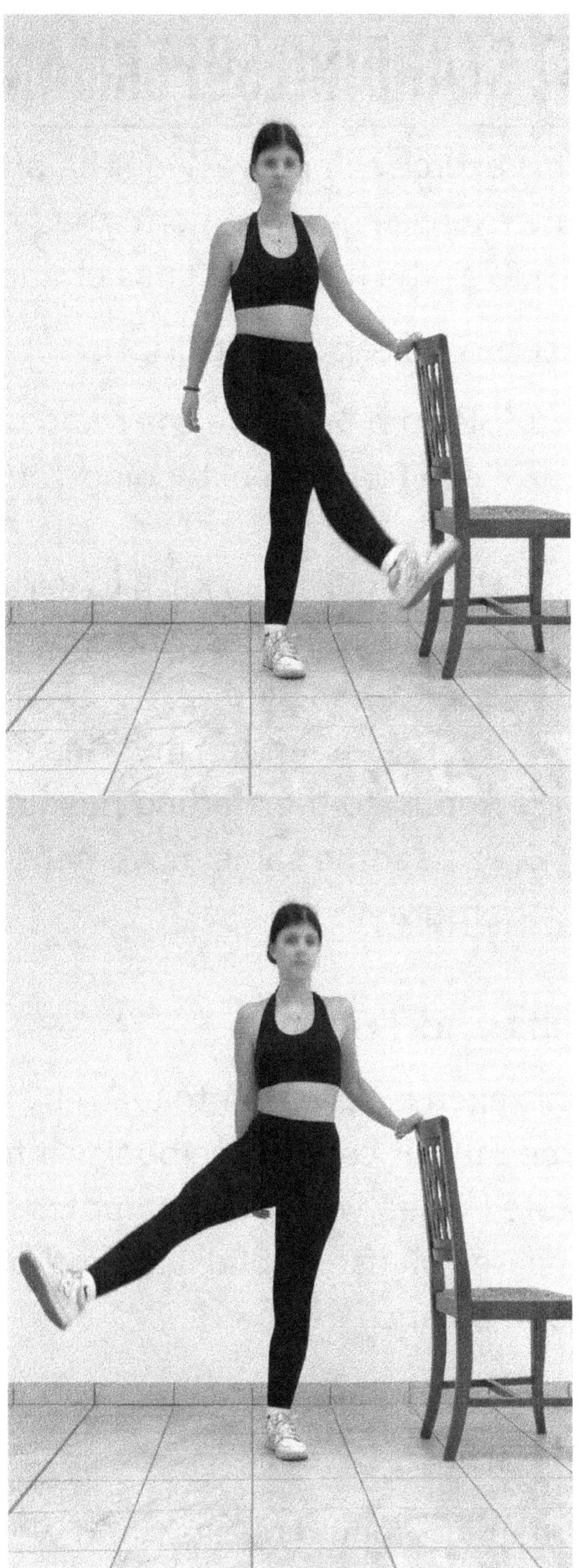

37 STANDING SUPERMAN POSE

This exercise improves your balance and tone your glute muscles. The exercise must be performed standing with the support of a chair. It makes the movement easier and safer while still being effective.

Step by Step Instructions

1. Stand behind the chair and place your left hand on the backrest
2. Lean forward, extending your right leg back and raising your right arm
3. Raise your torso back to vertical while bringing your right knee toward your chest and to a 90° angle, and moving your right arm to your side
4. Keep your left leg muscles engaged during the entire movement
5. Return to the starting position
6. Repeat the same movement based on the frequency in the daily program

Tips and Tricks

This exercise is easier to learn by watching the companion videos (see the QR code in the book's introduction section). Contracting your glutes when you extend your leg backwards helps tone them faster. Ensure you use a solid, stable chair or the edge of a table to ensure good balance.

Breathing

Breathing should be slow and well-controlled.

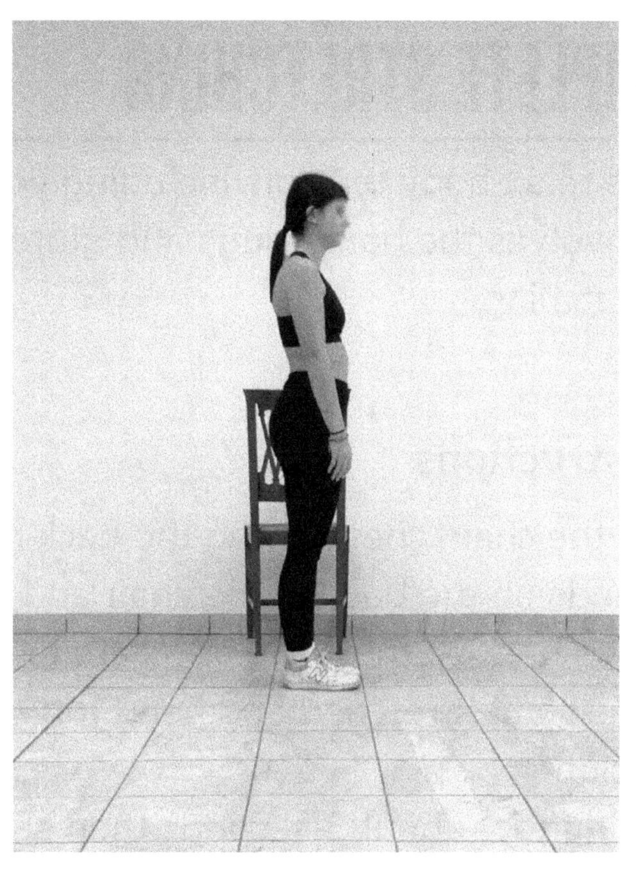

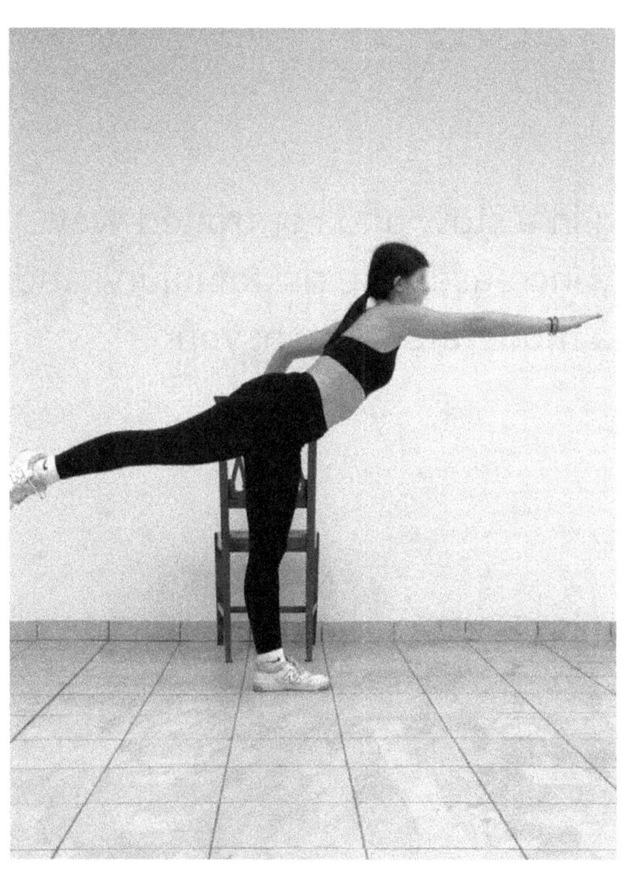

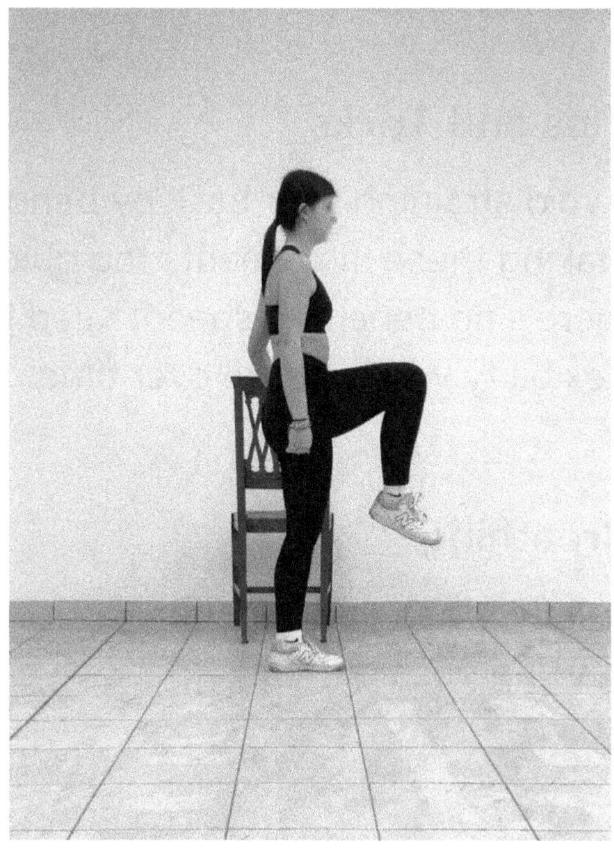

38 SPINE COMPLETE STRETCHING

This exercise helps relax body tension, including your back muscles. Moreover, it also involves the hamstrings and glutes to provide very comprehensive stretching.

Step by Step Instructions

1. Stand behind the chair, chest facing the back rest
2. Place your hands on the back of the chair and shuffle your feet 3-4 small steps back so that your arms are extended
3. Keep your legs semi-stretched and bend forward, keeping your and arms straight
4. Hold this position for about 3 seconds then stand back up
5. Repeat based on the frequency in the daily program

Tips and Tricks

Avoid straining your back by bending in a slow and controlled way. Making these movements too quickly increases the risk of injury, and there's no benefit to speed. Keep to a moderate stretch; your flexibility will increase over time.

Breathing

Exhale when you bend forward, inhale when you return to the starting position.

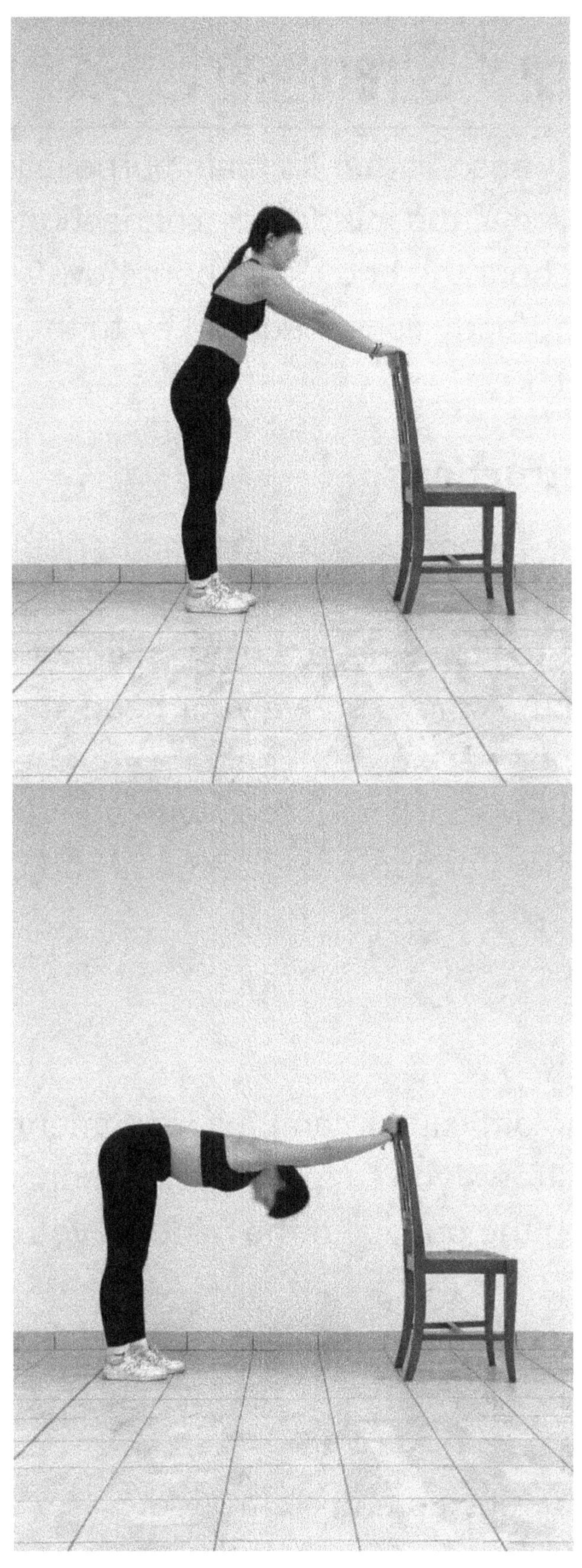

39 Praying Pose + Stretching

This is not a difficult pose, rather its main purpose is to relax your entire body and improve the mind/body connection. Feeling fit and healthy is not just about the body, it's about how we feel in our bodies, and the mind/body connection is key to that.

Step by Step Instructions

1. Sit on the chair, joining your hands and bending the elbows (see photo)
2. Move your out to your side, drawing an imaginary circle with your hands as they move above your head
3. Bring your hands back together above your head
4. Bend forward and touch your toes with your hands
5. Hold this position for about 2-3 seconds and then return to the starting position

Tips and Tricks

This exercise has no difficult or complex movements, making it easy to memorize. This allows you to focus your attention only on the connection between the body and the mind as you perform the movements.

Breathing

Keep your breathing relaxed and controlled.

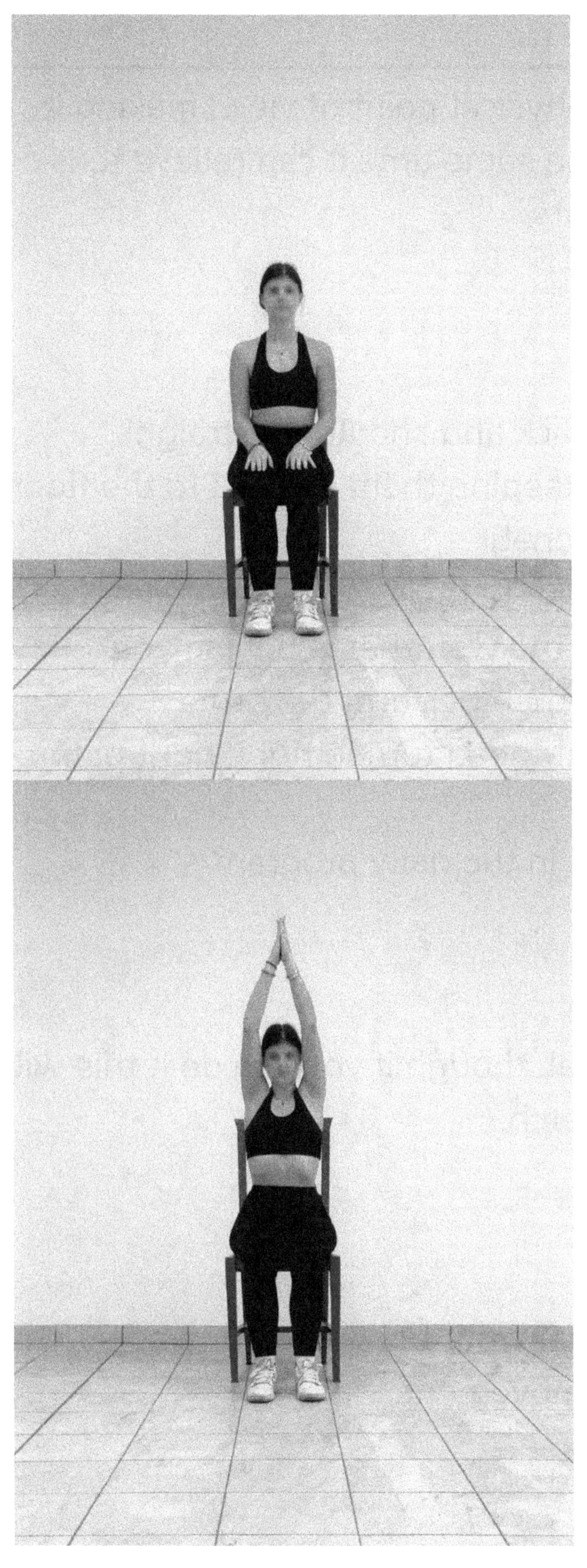

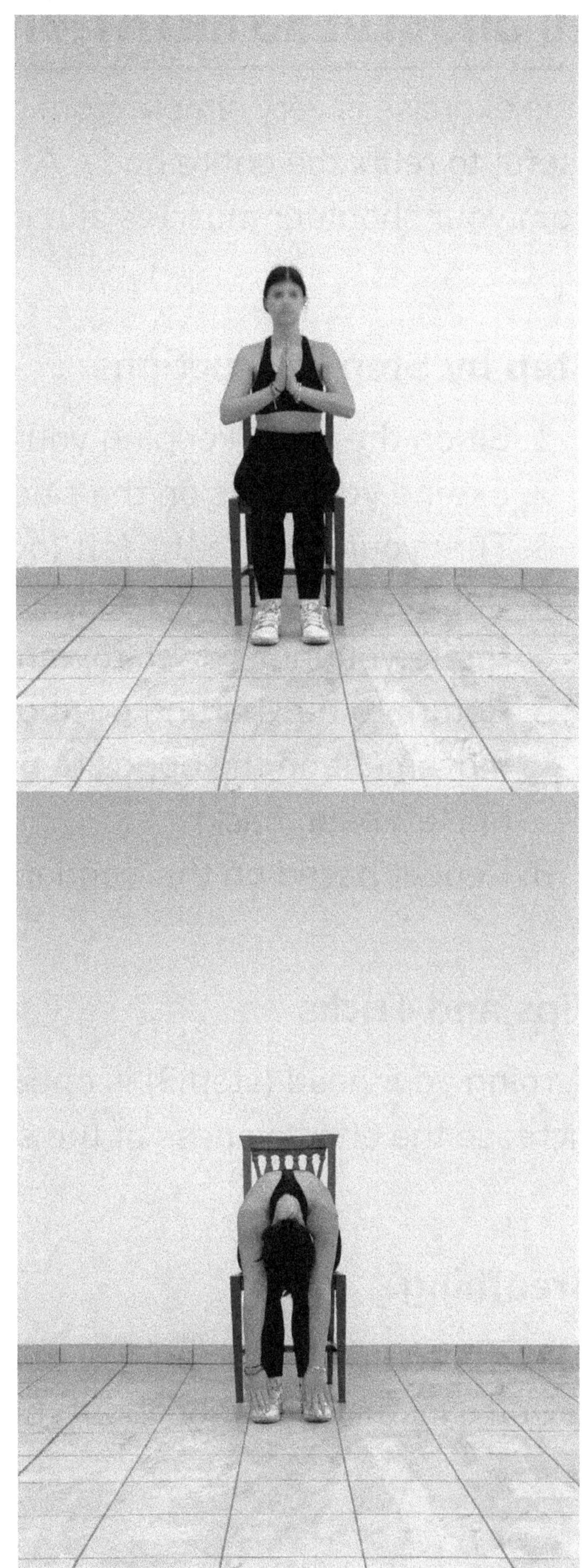

40 SHOULDERS ROTATION

This exercise is very simple from a physical point of view, making it useful to relax the entire body. At the same time it can relieve tension from your shoulder muscles and joints.

Step by Step Instructions

1. Sit on the chair, keeping your back and shoulders straight
2. Extend your arms on the side, keeping them parallel to the floor
3. Turn your head to the left (optional)
4. Rotate your left hand so that your palm is facing the ceiling, and rotate your right palm towards the wall that is behind you
5. Return to the starting position, then perform the same movement on the opposite right (head turned right, right palm up, left palm back)
6. Repeat based on the frequency in the daily program

Tips and Tricks

Turning your head (step 3) is optional, though if you can do it this will increase the effectiveness of the stretch.

Breathing

Keep controlled breathing. Try to relax your body and mind as much as you can, thinking only about the movement.

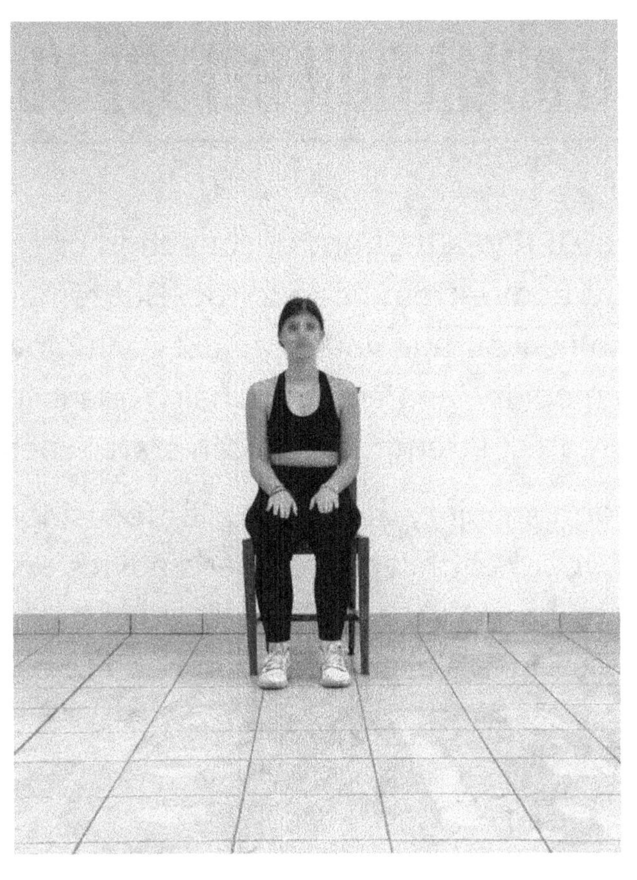

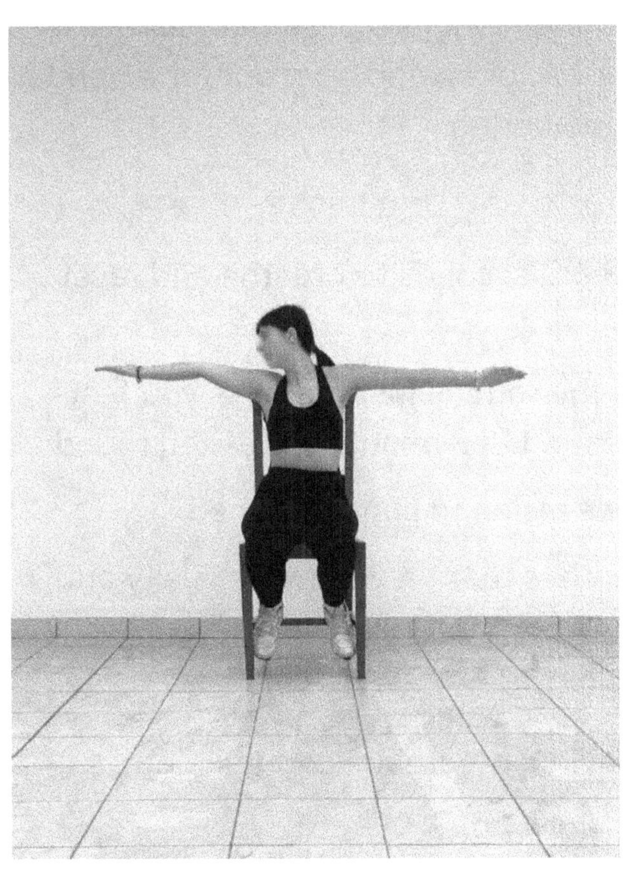

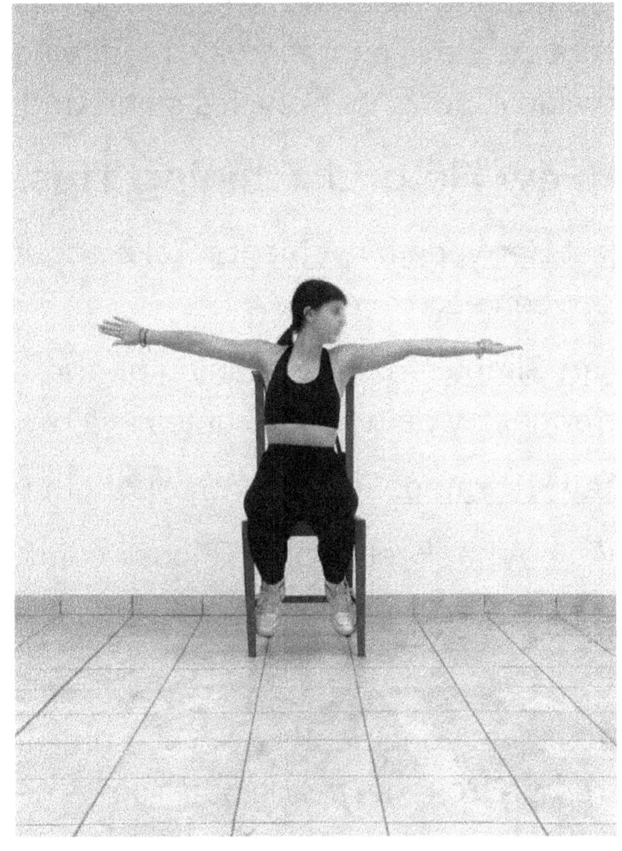

IMPORTANT INFORMATION BEFORE YOU START!

Within these pages you'll find a thoughtful collection of exercises designed to gently engage your full body—from head to toe. But remember, your body is wonderfully unique, so I encourage you to adjust each movement to suit your current comfort level, mobility, and energy. Chair Yoga is incredibly adaptable, and that's one of its greatest strengths; you can start exactly where you are.

If you're working through an injury, recovering, or focusing on specific areas, it's always best to follow your healthcare provider's advice and choose exercises from this program that support your healing. If you're beginning with a general level of fitness, this guide offers everything you need to confidently start your Chair Yoga journey.

Listen to Your Body

This is your time. So, please check in with your body often during each session. If something feels too difficult or doesn't quite work for you, don't push—there's always another way. Modifying a move or swapping it out for a gentler version is not only okay, it's smart and empowering.

A Few Helpful Training Tips:

Rest Between Movements: Take about 60–90 seconds to breathe and reset between each exercise.

Start Simple: In the beginning go through the routine just once. As you feel stronger try doing it 2–3 times in a row, resting 2–3 minutes between rounds.

Stay Hydrated: Sip water throughout your session to stay refreshed.

Wear What Feels Good: Choose comfy clothes that let you move easily and feel good on your skin.

Let's take it one gentle step at a time—moving, breathing, and building strength from the inside out. You've got this.

28-DAY FAT BURNING PROGRAM

DAY 1:

DATE: _______________

EXERCISE	PAGE	REPETITIONS/DURATION	✓
1	1	5 REPETITIONS PER SIDE	
5	9	5 REPETITIONS PER LEG	
7	13	5 REPETITIONS PER SIDE	
23	45	5 REPETITIONS PER LEG	
40	79	5 REPETITIONS PER SIDE	
34	67	10 REPETITIONS	

(The last column of the table is for you; you can use a pen to mark every time you complete the exercise)

DAY 2

DATE: _______________

EXERCISE	PAGE	REPETITIONS/DURATION	✓
2	3	5 REPETITIONS PER ARM	
6	11	10 REPETITIONS	
8	15	5 REPETITIONS PER LEG	
23	45	5 REPETITIONS PER LEG	
32	63	5 REPETITIONS PER SIDE	
15	29	5 REPETITIONS PER LEG	

DAY 3

DATE: _____________

EXERCISE	PAGE	REPETITIONS/DURATION	✓
3	5	10 REPETITIONS	
9	17	5 REPETITIONS PER LEG	
11	21	10 REPETITIONS	
25	49	5 REPETITIONS	
38	75	10 REPETITIONS	
16	31	10 REPETITIONS	

DAY 4

DATE: _____________

EXERCISE	PAGE	REPETITIONS/DURATION	✓
4	7	5 REPETITIONS PER SIDE	
10	19	10 REPETITIONS	
12	23	10 REPETITIONS	
26	51	5 REPETITIONS PER SIDE	
39	77	10 REPETITIONS	
17	33	5 REPETITIONS PER LEG	

DAY 5

DATE: ________________

EXERCISE	PAGE	REPETITIONS/DURATION	✔
13	25	10 REPETITIONS	
14	27	15 REPETITIONS	
18	35	5 REPETITIONS PER SIDE	
27	53	5 REPETITIONS PER SIDE	
35	69	5 REPETITIONS PER LEG	
19	37	5 REPETITIONS PER SIDE	

DAY 6

DATE: ________________

EXERCISE	PAGE	REPETITIONS/DURATION	✔
20	39	5 REPETITIONS PER LEG	
28	55	5 REPETITIONS PER LEG	
36	71	5 REPETITIONS PER LEG	
39	77	10 REPETITIONS	
24	47	5 REPETITIONS PER LEG	
21	41	5 REPETITIONS PER SIDE	

DAY 7

DATE: _______________

EXERCISE	PAGE	REPETITIONS/DURATION	✓
22	43	10 REPETITIONS	
29	57	5 REPETITIONS PER SIDE	
37	73	5 REPETITIONS PER LEG	
40	79	5 REPETITIONS PER SIDE	
30	59	5 REPETITIONS PER SIDE	
33	65	5 REPETITIONS PER SIDE	

DAY 8

DATE: _______________

EXERCISE	PAGE	REPETITIONS/DURATION	✓
31	61	10 REPETITIONS	
38	75	10 REPETITIONS	
15	29	5 REPETITIONS PER LEG	
24	47	5 REPETITIONS PER LEG	
21	41	5 REPETITIONS PER SIDE	
39	77	10 REPETITIONS	

DAY 9

DATE: _______________

EXERCISE	PAGE	REPETITIONS/DURATION	✓
22	43	10 REPETITIONS	
30	59	5 REPETITIONS PER SIDE	
33	65	5 REPETITIONS PER SIDE	
1	1	5 REPETITIONS PER SIDE	
36	71	5 REPETITIONS PER LEG	
15	29	5 REPETITIONS PER LEG	

DAY 10

DATE: _______________

EXERCISE	PAGE	REPETITIONS/DURATION	✓
11	21	10 REPETITIONS	
16	31	10 REPETITIONS	
19	37	5 REPETITIONS PER SIDE	
25	49	5 REPETITIONS	
32	63	5 REPETITIONS PER SIDE	
37	73	5 REPETITIONS PER LEG	

DAY 11

DATE: _______________

EXERCISE	PAGE	REPETITIONS/DURATION	✓
13	25	10 REPETITIONS	
18	35	5 REPETITIONS PER SIDE	
27	53	5 REPETITIONS PER SIDE	
35	69	5 REPETITIONS PER LEG	
19	37	5 REPETITIONS PER SIDE	
40	79	5 REPETITIONS PER SIDE	

DAY 12

DATE: _______________

EXERCISE	PAGE	REPETITIONS/DURATION	✓
20	39	5 REPETITIONS PER LEG	
28	55	5 REPETITIONS PER LEG	
36	71	5 REPETITIONS PER LEG	
38	75	10 REPETITIONS	
24	47	5 REPETITIONS PER LEG	
21	41	5 REPETITIONS PER SIDE	

DAY 13

DATE: _____________

EXERCISE	PAGE	REPETITIONS/DURATION	✓
22	43	10 REPETITIONS	
29	57	5 REPETITIONS PER SIDE	
37	73	5 REPETITIONS PER LEG	
2	3	5 REPETITIONS PER ARM	
30	59	5 REPETITIONS PER SIDE	
33	65	5 REPETITIONS PER SIDE	

DAY 14

DATE: _____________

EXERCISE	PAGE	REPETITIONS/DURATION	✓
31	61	10 REPETITIONS	
5	9	5 REPETITIONS PER LEG	
16	31	10 REPETITIONS	
24	47	5 REPETITIONS PER LEG	
21	41	5 REPETITIONS PER SIDE	
39	77	10 REPETITIONS	

DAY 15

DATE: _______________

EXERCISE	PAGE	REPETITIONS/DURATION	✓
22	43	10 REPETITIONS	
30	59	5 REPETITIONS PER SIDE	
33	65	5 REPETITIONS PER SIDE	
8	15	5 REPETITIONS PER LEG	
36	71	5 REPETITIONS PER LEG	
1	1	5 REPETITIONS PER SIDE	

DAY 16

DATE: _______________

EXERCISE	PAGE	REPETITIONS/DURATION	✓
11	21	10 REPETITIONS	
16	31	10 REPETITIONS	
19	37	5 REPETITIONS PER SIDE	
25	49	5 REPETITIONS	
32	63	5 REPETITIONS PER SIDE	
12	23	10 REPETITIONS	

DAY 17

DATE: ________________

EXERCISE	PAGE	REPETITIONS/DURATION	✓
13	25	10 REPETITIONS	
18	35	5 REPETITIONS PER SIDE	
27	53	5 REPETITIONS PER SIDE	
35	69	5 REPETITIONS PER LEG	
19	37	5 REPETITIONS PER SIDE	
30	59	5 REPETITIONS PER SIDE	

DAY 18

DATE: ________________

EXERCISE	PAGE	REPETITIONS/DURATION	✓
20	39	5 REPETITIONS PER LEG	
28	55	5 REPETITIONS PER LEG	
36	71	5 REPETITIONS PER LEG	
3	5	10 REPETITIONS	
24	47	5 REPETITIONS PER LEG	
21	41	5 REPETITIONS PER SIDE	

DAY 19

DATE: _______________

EXERCISE	PAGE	REPETITIONS/DURATION	✓
22	43	10 REPETITIONS	
29	57	5 REPETITIONS PER SIDE	
37	73	5 REPETITIONS PER LEG	
9	17	5 REPETITIONS PER LEG	
30	59	5 REPETITIONS PER SIDE	
33	65	5 REPETITIONS PER SIDE	

DAY 20

DATE: _______________

EXERCISE	PAGE	REPETITIONS/DURATION	✓
31	61	10 REPETITIONS	
12	23	10 REPETITIONS	
16	31	10 REPETITIONS	
24	47	5 REPETITIONS PER LEG	
21	41	5 REPETITIONS PER SIDE	
39	77	10 REPETITIONS	

DAY 21

DATE: _______________

EXERCISE	PAGE	REPETITIONS/DURATION	✓
22	43	10 REPETITIONS	
30	59	5 REPETITIONS PER SIDE	
33	65	5 REPETITIONS PER SIDE	
5	9	5 REPETITIONS PER LEG	
36	71	5 REPETITIONS PER LEG	
8	15	5 REPETITIONS PER LEG	

DAY 22

DATE: _______________

EXERCISE	PAGE	REPETITIONS/DURATION	✓
11	21	10 REPETITIONS	
16	31	10 REPETITIONS	
19	37	5 REPETITIONS PER SIDE	
25	49	5 REPETITIONS	
32	63	5 REPETITIONS PER SIDE	
15	29	5 REPETITIONS PER LEG	

DAY 23

DATE: _______________

EXERCISE	PAGE	REPETITIONS/DURATION	✓
13	25	10 REPETITIONS	
18	35	5 REPETITIONS PER SIDE	
27	53	5 REPETITIONS PER SIDE	
35	69	5 REPETITIONS PER LEG	
19	37	5 REPETITIONS PER SIDE	
6	11	10 REPETITIONS	

DAY 24

DATE: _______________

EXERCISE	PAGE	REPETITIONS/DURATION	✓
20	39	5 REPETITIONS PER LEG	
28	55	5 REPETITIONS PER LEG	
36	71	5 REPETITIONS PER LEG	
1	1	5 REPETITIONS PER SIDE	
24	47	5 REPETITIONS PER LEG	
15	29	5 REPETITIONS PER LEG	

DAY 25

DATE: _______________

EXERCISE	PAGE	REPETITIONS/DURATION	✓
22	43	10 REPETITIONS	
29	57	5 REPETITIONS PER SIDE	
37	73	5 REPETITIONS PER LEG	
4	7	5 REPETITIONS PER SIDE	
30	59	5 REPETITIONS PER SIDE	
33	65	5 REPETITIONS PER SIDE	

DAY 26

DATE: _______________

EXERCISE	PAGE	REPETITIONS/DURATION	✓
31	61	10 REPETITIONS	
38	75	10 REPETITIONS	
9	17	5 REPETITIONS PER LEG	
24	47	5 REPETITIONS PER LEG	
21	41	5 REPETITIONS PER SIDE	
39	77	10 REPETITIONS	

DAY 27

DATE: _______________

EXERCISE	PAGE	REPETITIONS/DURATION	✓
22	43	10 REPETITIONS	
30	59	5 REPETITIONS PER SIDE	
33	65	5 REPETITIONS PER SIDE	
15	29	5 REPETITIONS PER LEG	
36	71	5 REPETITIONS PER LEG	
10	19	10 REPETITIONS	

DAY 28

DATE: _______________

EXERCISE	PAGE	REPETITIONS/DURATION	✓
11	21	10 REPETITIONS	
16	31	10 REPETITIONS	
19	37	5 REPETITIONS PER SIDE	
25	49	5 REPETITIONS	
32	63	5 REPETITIONS PER SIDE	
8	15	5 REPETITIONS PER LEG	

TRACKING CHART

DAY	WORKOUT DURATION	MOTIVATION (HIGH/LOW)	ARE YOU PROUD OF YOUR SELF?
DAY 1			
DAY 2			
DAY 3			
DAY 4			
DAY 5			
DAY 6			
DAY 7			
DAY 8			
DAY 9			
DAY 10			

DAY	WORKOUT DURATION	MOTIVATION (HIGH/LOW)	ARE YOU PROUD OF YOUR SELF?
DAY 11			
DAY 12			
DAY 13			
DAY 14			
DAY 15			
DAY 16			
DAY 17			
DAY 18			
DAY 19			
DAY 20			
DAY 21			

DAY	WORKOUT DURATION	MOTIVATION (HIGH/LOW)	ARE YOU PROUD OF YOUR SELF?
DAY 22			
DAY 23			
DAY 24			
DAY 25			
DAY 26			
DAY 27			
DAY 28